YOGABODY

By Judith Hanson Lasater, Ph.D., PT

Relax and Renew

Living Your Yoga

30 Essential Yoga Poses

Yoga for Pregnancy

Yoga Abs

A Year of Living Your Yoga

Yogabody

What We Say Matters
(with Ike K. Lasater)

Yogabody

ANATOMY, KINESIOLOGY, AND ASANA

Judith Hanson Lasater, Ph.D., P.T.

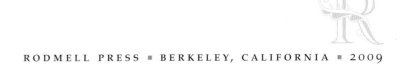

RODMELL PRESS ▪ BERKELEY, CALIFORNIA ▪ 2009

No part of this book may be reproduced or transmitted in any form or by any means, electronic or mechanical, including photocopying, recording, or by an information storage or retrieval system, without written permission from Rodmell Press, 2147 Blake St., Berkeley, CA 94704-2715; (510) 841-3123, (510) 841-3191 (fax), www.rodmellpress.com.

Library of Congress Cataloging-in-Publication Data
Lasater, Judith.
Yogabody : anatomy, kinesiology, and asana / Judith Hanson Lasater. — 1st ed.   p. cm.
Includes bibliographical references and index. ISBN 978-1-930485-21-1 (pbk. : alk. paper) — ISBN 978-1-930485-23-5 (hardcover : alk. paper)
1. Hatha yoga. I. Title. II. Title: Yoga body.
RA781.7.L375 2009
613.7'046—dc22
                                    2008052134

Printed and bound in China
First edition
Hardcover: ISBN-13: 978-1-930485-23-5
Trade Paper: ISBN-13: 978-1-930485-21-1
17 16 15 14 13   5 6 7 8 9 10

Editor: Linda Cogozzo
Associate Editor: Holly Hammond
Indexer: Ty Koontz
Design: Gopa & Ted2, Inc.
Anatomy Illustrations: Sharon Ellis and Lauren Keswick
Asana Illustrations: Sharon Ellis
Cover Photograph: David Martinez, Inc.
Lithographer: Kwong Fat Offset Printing Co., Ltd.
Text set in Palatino LT Std 9.8/14.6

Distributed by Publishers Group West

To Charles Kampmann Lasater

Contents

Acknowledgments

MORE THAN MOST people realize, writing a book requires the support of a number of people. This book has been particularly shaped by two people. The first is my son, Charles Kampmann "Kam" Lasater and the second is Dr. Ruth Williams.

Years ago I was preparing to travel for the second time to India to study yoga with my teacher. Plans had been set for a year, and I was excited each time I thought about the trip. However, on our first son's second birthday, we learned that a second baby was coming. I cancelled my trip, and at the suggestion of my husband, I spent the time I had set aside writing the outline of an anatomy and kinesiology book. I used those outlines frequently as the basis for articles and workshops through the years. Now I am finally fulfilling a life's dream by writing the book I planned so many years ago. Because of Kam, I began this book more than two decades ago. For his part in its creation, and for the joy his life has brought me, I am so grateful.

The other person who helped shape this book has shared her talents for months, doing the not-so-exciting work of reading and helping with the manuscript. Ruth Williams started her life's work as an artist. Her next project was raising three daughters. As they grew up, she reconnected with an early love of science, returning to school to study biology and chemistry. Upon graduation she received a research and teaching fellowship in gross anatomy and neuroanatomy at the University of Tennessee School of Medicine, where she completed a doctorate in anatomy.

However, I did not meet Dr. Williams in an anatomy class but in a yoga class. She was participating in a teacher training I was giving. In addition to her teaching of anatomy, she had become a yoga teacher. We instantly connected around our love of the two disciplines, and within a matter of hours I had asked her to help me with this book. I appreciate not only the competence but also the good nature with which she did so. The truth is that Dr. Williams has made this book a much better one, and we all benefit. I am deeply grateful.

My gratitude is also especially offered to Jill Jalaja Korengold, not only for the admirable and helpful job she did reading the completed manuscript but also for the work she does in the world. She has studied and taught yoga science since 1988 with the blessings of Sadguru Sant Keshavadas, Srimad Rama Mata, and Sri Haricharandas. In addition, she is a bilingual teacher of elementary students and shares her love and knowledge of yoga science with them.

I extend my appreciation to Angela Zaragoza,

D.C., and Athena Kyle, P.T., both of San Francisco, who answered my questions about anatomy and function whenever I asked, and did so graciously and competently every time.

I would also like to thank my publishers at Rodmell Press, Linda Cogozzo and Donald Moyer. This is our seventh book together, and I continue to enjoy our working relationship and treasure our friendship.

Finally, my family's support is always part of the writing of my books. My thanks and love to them.

Introduction:
The Shape of *Yogabody*

IF ANYTHING IS SACRED, THE HUMAN BODY IS SACRED.
—WALT WHITMAN

THE ANCIENT INDIAN philosophy of yoga has many schools of thought and a variety of techniques, the most popular of which is asana. The practice of asana has historically been taught to prepare the *sadhaka* (seeker) for the prolonged practices of meditation. Today, however, yoga asana is being used by millions of people throughout the world for other reasons as well: to reduce stress, improve health, enhance athletic performance, recover from injury and illness, as well as to simply improve the enjoyment of daily life.

As a result of this popularity, an increasing number of yoga teachers are teaching classes in all imaginable venues. This book is written for you. My goal is to offer to the experienced and the novice teacher a thorough presentation of the basic systems that create and control movement in the body. Furthermore, it is my wish to present this information in a manner that will render it immediately useful in your yoga studio class. This book is also

for you, the yoga student, to help you understand how your body functions so you can become your own teacher when practicing on your own. What follows is a brief explanation of the emphasis and organization of this book.

Anatomy is the study of the structure of the human body. To study anatomy, the structure of the organism, is like learning the letters of the alphabet, the basic building blocks of words. Kinesiology is the study of the movement of that body through space; to study kinesiology is to put those "letters" together to make the "words" of movement. You can't fully understand the dynamic movement of asana without first understanding the basic structure of the human body.

This book will focus on both anatomy and kinesiology in relationship to asana practice and teaching. By understanding the structure and function of the locomotor system, you will become a more effective and efficient practitioner and teacher. You will be better able to quickly decide what might be able to help you and your students move with more enjoyment and less difficulty or pain.

My emphasis is on macroanatomy, the anatomy of the major structures of the body. I do not discuss microanatomy, such as the structure of the cell or the specific fibers of muscles. I have written *Yogabody* as if I were teaching an anatomy class. My hope is twofold. The first is that this book will be a direct and friendly connection from me to you, and then of you to the subject matter. My second hope is that what you learn in the pages of *Yogabody* will be interesting and immediately applicable to your practice and teaching, not merely a collection of facts about the body. This book does not include all the details about the anatomy of the body, but it does, I hope, include enough to keep you interested and learning for a very long time.

HOW TO USE THIS BOOK

Yogabody is divided into five parts: the locomotor system, the vertebral column, the lower extremity, the trunk, and the upper extremity.

Each chapter focuses on a specific region of the body. In addition, there is a chapter each on the diaphragm and the abdomen, even though these areas are not as directly related to the locomotor system as is the vertebral column, for example. I include the diaphragm and abdomen because I feel it is useful for you to understand the structure of these parts of the body when teaching yoga asana. You will only benefit by knowing where all the abdominal organs are, their relationship one to another, and how these organs could be affected by the various positions, such as inversions.

Each chapter begins with an epigraph, a quote to enlighten and amuse. Then comes a section on the bones, which discusses the bony structures of the area, including any specific and unusual aspects found there. Next we look at the joints, the pertinent connective tissue, the nerves, and the muscles. A discussion of the kinesiology of the area follows. Here we explore how anatomical structures interact to create and express movement, especially in asana.

The final part of each chapter is called Experimental Anatomy. It has two sections that integrate the information presented in the previous two sections of anatomy and kinesiology as they relate to asana. The first, For Practicing, outlines one or more movements you can explore on your own to further your understanding of the principles presented in the chapter. For Teaching offers points to use and look for when teaching asana. The names and alignments suggested in these sections are based on the poses and approach of B. K. S. Iyengar of Pune, India, author of *Light on Yoga* and other books.

Each chapter concludes with Links, a section that offers connections for further learning.

My wish is that this book will become not only a guide but also a friend, to be consulted time and again to enrich and enhance your practice and teaching. May you read it with enthusiasm and curiosity.

Bones, Joints, Ligaments, Tendons, and Nerves 1

THE PROPERTIES OF THE SOUL DEPEND ON THE CONDITION OF THE BODY.

—MOSES MAIMONIDES

MY INTEREST IN ANATOMY began in seventh grade science class. That interest has deepened not only by my practice of yoga but also by my study of physical therapy. Overwhelmed by course work in physical therapy school and hoping to cut down on our study time, we students would plead with our anatomy teacher, Just how much do we have to know? Her answer was always the same: Know everything. Our response was always the same: a loud groan.

But really there are no useless details in the study of anatomy. Learn as much as you can. Make it a lifetime inquiry. I predict that it will enrich your personal asana practice. Even if we as yoga teachers never "know everything," that which we do know will help us teach in ways that prevent injury and enhance practice.

The locomotor system consists of several smaller systems, the bones and joints, as well as soft tissue like connective tissue, nerves, and muscles, which all work together to help us locomote, or move.

BONES

The underlying structure that allows the human body to move is the skeleton, a collection of 206 individual bones. The skeleton is divided into two main parts: the axial and the appendicular. The axial skeleton is made of the bones that form the axis of the human body: the skull and vertebral column, the ribs and sternum, and the hyoid bone, seventy-four in number. The appendicular skeleton consists of the limbs, or the arms and the legs. These number sixty-four in the upper extremity and sixty-two in the lower extremity. Adding six more auditory ossicles makes a grand total of 206 bones.

Each bone is made up of a vascular covering called a periosteum, which is painful to firm touch. This is not a surprise to anyone who has banged his shin on a table; that is periosteal pain. Bone is one-third living tissue and is basically a protein matrix with various minerals like calcium and

5

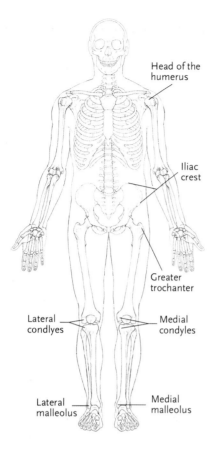

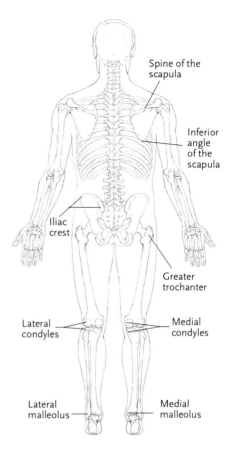

Labels on figure 1.1 (anterior view):
Head of the humerus
Iliac crest
Greater trochanter
Lateral condlyes
Medial condyles
Lateral malleolus
Medial malleolus

Labels on figure 1.2 (posterior view):
Spine of the scapula
Inferior angle of the scapula
Iliac crest
Greater trochanter
Lateral condyles
Medial condyles
Lateral malleolus
Medial malleolus

1.1 SKELETON, WITH BONY PROMINENCES AND THREE PLANES, ANTERIOR VIEW

1.2 SKELETON, WITH BONY PROMINENCES, POSTERIOR VIEW

other inorganic salts embedded in it. The marrow, found at the center of the large bones, is one of the sites that produce red blood cells. (The other is the spleen.) The function of red blood cells is to carry oxygen in the bloodstream.

At the end of each long bone is an epiphysis, or growth plate: this is exactly what it sounds like. Bones grow from their ends, and when an individual has reached her maturity, the growth plates are no longer active.

Another function of bone is to act as a storage place for minerals, such as calcium. When calcium is needed for a variety of physiological functions in the body, it can be released from the bones to that service.

Wolfe's law states that bones grow along lines of stress. This means that when we bear weight on our bones, especially on those that are intended for weight bearing, such as the femur, it helps to strengthen the bone. Astronauts who have been weightless in space actually have lost a small percentage of their bone mass when they are tested back on Earth. Gravity causes weight to be borne through the bones, thus stimulating the bone to maintain itself.

Each bone is uniquely shaped to perform a specific function and may be described as long, short, or irregular. We will be mostly concerned with the major weight-bearing bones that are used in the practice of asana. Figures 1.1 and 1.2 show the front and back of the skeleton, known as the anterior and posterior views.

It is worthwhile, if not imperative, for a yoga teacher to memorize the names of all the bones.

Take the time to do that now. It can be useful when teaching yoga to be able to quickly touch various bony prominences, or anatomical markers, on the student's body. The following seven prominences are especially important to know:

▶ head of the humerus: the top rounded part of the upper arm bone as is fits into the shoulder joint

▶ spine of the scapula: a horizontal ridge that divides the posterior surface of the bone

▶ inferior angle of the scapula: its position will help you ascertain your student's scapular position

▶ interior superior iliac crest: commonly known as the hip bone. It should be level, not only right to left but also front to back. The angle of this prominence can inform you about the curve in the student's lower back.

▶ greater trochanter: the prominence on the outer upper thigh and an extension of the neck of the femur. Noting the position of this prominence can tell you about the rotation of the student's thigh and whether the student is standing with a neutral rotation of the hip.

▶ tubercles at the inner and outer knee joint: the site of attachment of many muscles

▶ malleoli: the lateral and medial ankle bones can help you identify ankle alignment

Bones come in a variety of shapes: long, short, flat, or irregular. For example, the humerus is a long bone, and a tarsal bone is a short one; the ilium is a flat bone, and a vertebra is irregular.

A special kind of irregular bone is a sesamoid bone. This is a bone that develops in the tendon of a muscle. The benefits of a sesamoid bone are to offer protection to the tendon as it passes over the joint during movement, as well as to offer increased leverage and thus power on contraction. An example of a sesamoid bone is the patella, or kneecap. The kneecap develops during the first year of life in the tendon of the quadriceps muscle as it passes over the knee joint.

Bones can have ridges, called spines, or crests, which serve as the attachment point of muscles and other connective tissue; they can have openings called foramen (singular) or foramina (plural). These openings allow for the passage of other structures, like nerves and blood vessels. Bones also have projections, like the tuberosity of the humerus and the trochanter of the femur.

Joints

A joint is the site where two bones come together; it is also called an articulation. Joints are considered either semi-rigid, like the joints between the bones of the skull and the symphysis pubis, or movable, like the knee joint.

Movable joints are also called synovial joints. This means they have a capsule that covers the end of the bones where the two bones come together. They also have a synovial lining inside the capsule, which produces synovial fluid to keep the joint moist and healthy, thus promoting easy movement.

An interesting fact about joint capsules: they have no direct blood supply. This means that the tissue of the joint capsule is only nourished by the periosteum of the adjacent bones, of which the capsule is an outgrowth. And this nourishment is partly created by movement. The movement of joints during asana practice can thus help the joint capsule stay healthy. Synovial joints can be subject to a variety of diseases, including rheumatoid arthritis, in which the synovium proliferates pathologically and interferes with and limits joint function, misshapes the joint, and causes pain.

Movable joints can be further divided into four categories:

▶ gliding: This is a joint where one bone glides easily against another, such as the acromioclavicular joint at the shoulder and the tarsals of the ankle (Figure 1.3).

▶ uniaxial: There are two types: hinge and pivot. A hinge joint is one in which the two surfaces of the joint move around each other, like a simple hinge. One of the surfaces of the joint is concave and the other is convex. An example of a hinge joint is the elbow joint (Figure 1.4). In a pivot joint, one bone pivots around the other in one direction. One example of a pivot joint is the proximal radio-ulnar joint (Figure 1.5).

A word here about the knee joint and its incorrect categorization as a hinge joint: While it may appear that the knee joint is a hinge joint, this is not entirely true. While the knee joint does have a hingelike function, a gliding action as well as a rotational component occur there, so the knee is a

1.3 GLIDING JOINT

1.4 UNIAXIAL JOINT (HINGE)

1.5 UNIAXIAL JOINT (PIVOT)

hybrid joint. The knee joint is discussed further in chapter 9.

▶ biaxial: In this type of joint, there are two axes of movement, one for flexion and extension and one for adduction and abduction. There is no rotation allowed. An example is the metacarpo-phalangeal joints of the hand (Figure 1.6). Experiment with this. Firmly hold the root of your middle finger of your left hand, very close to the beginning of the finger, between the thumb and first finger of your right hand, so that you can see the back of your left hand. Now, while holding your left hand absolutely stable, try to move the long column of the left middle finger gently up and down and then side to side. This should happen easily, although the movements are small. Remember to keep your left hand absolutely still as you move. Now try to rotate your finger longitudinally. This will not work. This is the hallmark of a biaxial joint.

▶ multiaxial: In this joint, the axis of movement can change. There are two types. The first is a saddle joint, in which the bones come together just like

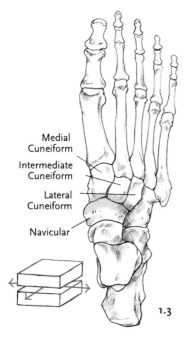

Medial Cuneiform
Intermediate Cuneiform
Lateral Cuneiform
Navicular

1.3

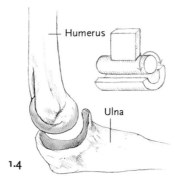

Humerus
Ulna

1.4

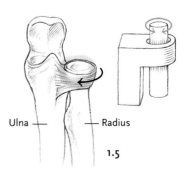

Ulna   Radius

1.5

a saddle fits on a horse. An example is the carpal joint of the thumb (Figure 1.7).

The other type is the ball-and-socket joint, such as the hip joint and the shoulder joint. They move in all directions: flexion, extension, adduction, abduction, and rotation. All these movements put together create circumduction (Figure 1.8).

CONNECTIVE TISSUE

By definition, connective tissue is any tissue that connects parts of the body. There are various types of connective tissue, ranging from hard (bone) to liquid (blood). They play important roles in the maintenance, protection, and anchoring of the skin, bones, and organs. For purposes of this book, we consider only the connective tissue that pertains directly to locomotion.

Bone is the hardest form of connective tissue. Cartilage is the form of connective tissue that serves a protective function, padding areas where use is great to prevent damage to bone. There are three types of cartilage:

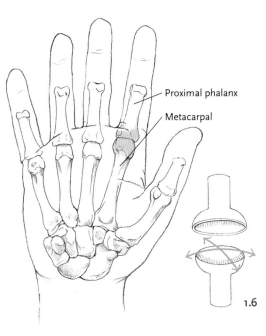

Proximal phalanx

Metacarpal

1.6

1.6 BIAXIAL JOINT

1.7 MULTIAXIAL JOINT

1.8 MULTIAXIAL JOINT, WITH SYNOVIUM AND CARTILAGE

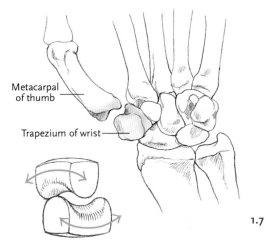

Metacarpal of thumb

Trapezium of wrist

1.7

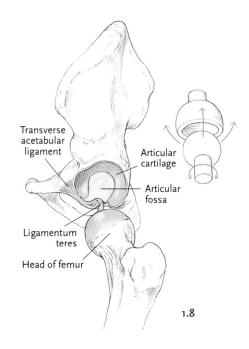

Transverse acetabular ligament

Articular cartilage

Articular fossa

Ligamentum teres

Head of femur

1.8

▶ fibro cartilage: This is a very dense material and makes up the symphysis pubis and the intervertebral discs.

▶ hyaline cartilage: This is more elastic than fibro cartilage and has the smooth consistency of hard, dense but bendable rubber. It is mainly found at the ends of bones. It attaches the lower ribs to the sternum and makes up most of the nose.

▶ elastic cartilage: Just as its names implies, this is the most elastic of all three types of cartilage, and the perfect example is the outer ear. It can also be found in small amounts in parts of the inner ear and larynx.

Fascia is another form of connective tissue. The superficial type is just under the skin. The deep fascia holds each muscle and can hold muscle groups as well. It is thin, white, and has a strong cobweb-like look. It also can serve as an anchor for the passage of nerves and blood vessels. After injury, the fascia can become adhered to surrounding tissues and interfere with pure muscle function and locomotion.

During asana practice, you may have noticed areas or specific muscles of your body that never seem to stretch out. The sensation of stretching that part of your body seems to be the same year after year. This could be an area where your fascia is adhered to surrounding tissue. You may find that a session or more of deep tissue work or massage can help to free up these areas when repeated asana practice cannot.

Ligaments are the form of connective tissue that holds bone to bone at every articulation. They are distensible but not very elastic. In other words, ligaments can be stretched from their original length; this can happen slowly over time with asana practice or quickly when one falls and sprains an ankle.

However, ligaments are not very elastic. This means that a strongly stretched or sprained ligament will not go back fully to its original shape, which is what the word *elastic* means. Think of a rubber band; it always goes back to its original shape when you pull it out. Ligaments do not (Figure 1.9).

Anyone who has sprained an ankle knows that the ligaments on the outside of that ankle are always a little looser than those on the outside of the ankle that has not been sprained. This low amount of elasticity is one of the factors that allow us to stay stretched out over time. Otherwise, every asana practice would feel like the very first one.

Tendons are the connective tissue that holds muscles to bones. The fibers of the muscle tendons are arranged in long, straight lines. The tendon grows out of the periosteum of one bone, goes through and around the muscle, and then attaches at the other end to the bone. Tendons are named for the muscle of which they are a part.

Bursae are sacs of connective tissue that have a synovial lining and secrete synovial fluid for ease of movement. Bursae are located at points in the body where movement creates friction and thus heat; they are primarily protective of tendons and muscles where they can rub over bones. Well-known bursae are located at the subacromial joint of the shoulder, the subdeltoid region, in the anterior shoulder joint to protect the long head of the biceps brachii, at the ischial tuberosity, and at the back of the knee joint. All these areas are areas of regular friction of tendons over bones.

NERVES

Nerves are one of the main communicating structures of the human body. (Hormones are another example.) The nervous system can be divided into several parts. The central nervous system (CNS) consists of the brain and spinal cord and is partly under conscious control. The peripheral nervous system (PNS) consists of motor nerves (movement), which leave the spinal cord carrying impulses for movement, and sensory nerves (sensation), which return information to the spinal cord and brain.

The autonomic nervous system (ANS) is not under voluntary control. The ANS controls the heart and other organs, including smooth muscle in the digestive and reproductive tracts, as well as activities in other glands. The ANS consists of the sympathetic division (SNS), which is responsible for activities that help us in the flight-or-fight mode, and the parasympathetic nervous system (PSNS), which controls activities of regeneration and assimilation. The PSNS consists mainly of the long vagus nerve, which leaves the brain and travels distally (away from the center of the body) near the spinal cord. The word *vagus* is related to the word *vagabond.* It is aptly named, because the vagus nerve travels throughout the torso, helping to control nonvoluntary functions. The PSNS is what is stimulated when we practice Savasana or other restorative yoga poses.

A typical voluntary motor nerve that helps us to move in asana is a part of the spinal nerves that exit on either side of the back all along the vertebral column (Figure 1.10). A spinal nerve has two parts: a posterior, or dorsal, root, which is the sensory portion, and the anterior, or ventral, root, which is the motor portion.

These nerves, as do all peripheral nerves, have a fatty insulating covering called myelin, a grayish sheath whose function is to conduct the nervous impulse through the body. Myelin evolved in mammals to speed nerve impulses through long appendages. Otherwise the impulse might take too much time to travel down the appendage, and the mammal would not be able to react quickly enough to prevent injury by moving or avoiding danger.

Multiple sclerosis (MS) is a disease that attacks this myelin sheath, thus making nerve transmission difficult or impossible. What we call polio is actually termed anterior horn cell poliomyelitis, so called because the virus that causes it attacks

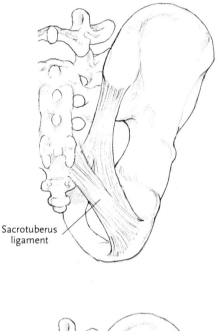

Sacrotuberus ligament

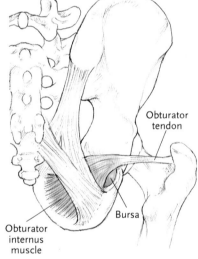

Obturator tendon

Obturator internus muscle

Bursa

1.9 (TOP) TENDON ATTACHED TO MUSCLE AND BONE, AND (BOTTOM) A LIGAMENT WITH BURSA

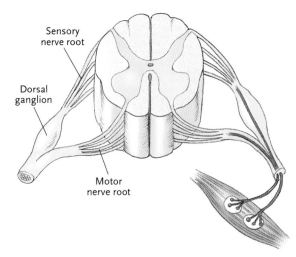

1.10 NERVE, WITH NEUROMUSCULAR JUNCTION

the anterior horn cell of the spinal column and destroys the motor root, thus causing paralysis of the limbs.

Locomotion is controlled not only by the peripheral motor nerves but also by various portions of the brain, such as the cerebellum, which is located at the back of the brain stem and is concerned with the unconscious coordination of muscle activity. A detailed discussion of such structures is beyond the scope of this book. However, a discussion of the specific motor nerves that control the movement of each section of the body can be found in their respective chapters.

MUSCLES

Muscles function to maintain our posture and to help us move. They give shape to the body and produce heat that helps to keep us warm. Muscles also help to hold the organs in place, and certain muscles help to open passageways in organs, allowing for the movement of food and digestive enzymes, the expulsion of solid and liquid waste, and the delivery of a baby and its placenta. Muscles are responsible for a large part of the functioning of the circulatory system, as well as for respiration and cardiac function.

There are three types of muscles in the body. These are smooth, or involuntary, muscles; cardiac muscle; and the skeletal, or voluntary, muscles, which most people think of when they think of their muscles.

Smooth muscle tissue is found in the walls of the stomach, intestines, uterus, arteries, arterioles, and bladder. Cardiac muscle tissue is found only in the walls of the heart. The skeletal or voluntary muscles are what we use to move the body. They give shape to our frame and hold us upright. In this book our focus is on skeletal muscles. Understanding the actions of these muscles is critical to understanding how to practice asana well and how to teach it with clarity and insight.

Muscles work by contracting, or shortening, and they also control movement when they release, or let go. The shortening is called a concentric contraction; I call it a shortening contraction. A muscle release can be sudden and swift, which is usually done in order to protect the muscle from tearing. However, most of the time muscles let go, or lengthen, in a slow and controlled manner. If a muscle lets go slowly, it is said to be undergoing an eccentric, or lengthening, contraction. While the term "lengthening contraction" may sound confusing, the principle is simple.

Try this experiment. Pick up something with about the weight of a hardback book with your right hand. Now set it down. Notice that you let it down slowly; you did not suddenly drop it. To prevent this sudden dropping, the muscles of your arm let go of their contraction slowly, so that the object is set down gently and not harmed. Try the action again, and this time lightly touch your right biceps muscle with the fingers of your left hand. Even though the biceps brachii is a flexor of the elbow, it is acting here to control extension.

Think of lowering something down over a cliff; if you let go of the rope, the object falls suddenly. While you are controlling the descent of the object, you are still doing metabolic work; your muscles are quite active while they are slowly letting go of the weight. This slow, controlled lengthening is a lengthening contraction, and we use this form of contraction all day long in our daily activities, as well as in the practice of asana.

For example, when you are in Salamba Sirsasana and are moving your straight legs down to come out of the pose, you are using a lengthening contraction in the muscles of the back of the legs, the hamstrings. This type of slow relaxation of the contraction, or lengthening of the hamstrings, helps to control the action of coming down, in effect, shaping the action. Without the hamstring muscles acting like brakes on the legs, they would drop down too suddenly instead of being lowered slowly.

KINESIOLOGY

Joints move because muscles contract and move them. In order to move, the capsule and the ligaments around the joint must have a certain amount of laxity, or joint play. Joint play means that the structures are loose on one side of the joint to facilitate movement on the opposite side.

To understand this concept, look at the top of your sleeve. When your humerus is hanging down in Tadasana, the top of the sleeve is taut and the underside or armpit side is loose. When you lift your humerus over your head, the opposite occurs: the top of your sleeve is now wrinkled and the armpit side is stretched. This is similar to what happens around the joint. A certain amount of looseness, or joint play, is necessary in order to allow for normal movement. If both sides of the joint capsule are taut, movement is greatly impeded.

Remember the movement you tried with your right hand moving your left index finger in two directions as an example of a biaxial joint (described on page 8)? That movement was allowed because the soft tissue structures around the joint had a good amount of joint play.

There are several types of joint movements that occur during locomotion:

▸ active joint movement: This is the voluntary movement in a joint that we do all day long when we get up and walk, dance, or practice asana.

▸ passive joint movement: This movement occurs when someone else moves your arm. The joint still moves, but the muscles and other structures are not doing their job to protect the joint. Moving the humerus is a complicated action that requires a number of muscles to provide a variety of functions (more on this later), and when the arm is moved by someone else, these additional actions are lacking. Therefore I recommend that, as much as possible, encourage your students to move actively and do not move the body part for the student.

▸ accessory joint movement: This is the movement of another joint, not the main one in use, in order to help or facilitate the desired action—for example, the rotation of the clavicle during shoulder flexion. The movement of the clavicle is not voluntary, or active, but is totally necessary for the shoulder joint to function normally. In other words, I cannot decide to rotate my clavicle voluntarily like I can to flex my shoulder joint, but nevertheless this rotation must occur in order for me to move

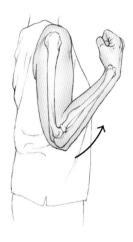

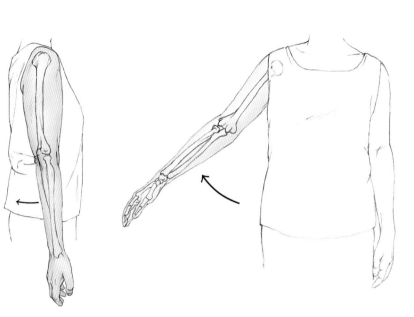

1.11 FLEXION OF A JOINT, RIGHT ELBOW

1.12 EXTENSION OF A JOINT, RIGHT ELBOW

1.13 ABDUCTION OF A JOINT, RIGHT ARM

my shoulder in a healthy way. This is discussed in detail in chapter 13, but you can feel it now.

With your left arm hanging down by your side, place the index and middle fingers of your right hand on your left clavicle where it is the most palpable. This point is between the sternum and humerus but a little closer to the sternum, where you feel the bone closest to the skin. Keep your right fingers in touch with your clavicle, and now raise your left arm out in front of you to shoulder height. You will feel your clavicle rotating backward under your fingers. Because you are unable to do this action voluntarily except as part of another action, in this case the flexing of the humerus, it is considered accessory joint movement.

Joints of the body move in specific ways, usually in pairs of opposites. The names of the movements are based on starting in anatomical position, such as is shown in illustrations at the beginning of this chapter. These movements are referred to by the joint name, not by the name of the bone.

Flexion is the reduction of an angle. An example of flexion is the bending of the elbow joint (Fig-

ure 1.11). We say, "flexion of the elbow joint" rather than "flexion of the ulna bone." Flexion of the vertebral column is to bend forward. Lateral flexion, or as I call it in this book, side bending, is a sideways bend of the vertebral column.

Extension means to straighten an angle (Figure 1.12). This is what happens when you straighten your arm, for example. It also means to back-bend the vertebral column. The term *hyperextension*, which means too much extension, or extension that is past an angle of 180 degrees, is considered pathological and is not a desired state for joints such as the elbow or knee.

Abduction is bringing a limb away from the midline (Figure 1.13). An example of abduction is to raise your upper extremity out to the side, as is done in standing poses. To adduct is to do the opposite: to bring the body part across the midline, as in reaching your arm across to your opposite leg to grasp the foot in Janu Sirsasana (Figure 1.14).

Rotation is the action of moving of a bone along its long axis. An example of internal rotation is what happens to the shoulder joint as you begin to put the arm behind the back in Namaste (Figure

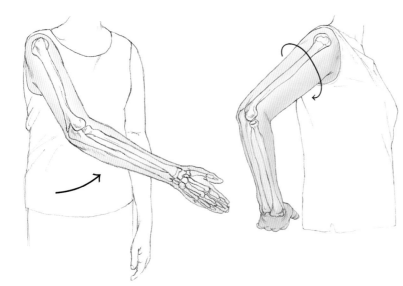

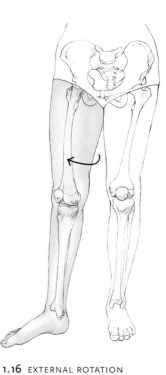

1.14 ADDUCTION OF A JOINT, RIGHT ARM

1.15 INTERNAL ROTATION OF A JOINT, RIGHT SHOULDER

1.16 EXTERNAL ROTATION OF A JOINT, RIGHT HIP

1.15). External rotation of a bone, for example the femur, occurs in Baddha Konasana (Figure 1.16).

Circumduction is the combination of flexion, extension, abduction, and adduction in sequence, such as moving the shoulder joint in large circles.

Supination and pronation are special movements of the hands and ankles. To supinate at the

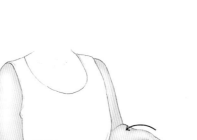

1.17 SUPINATION, LEFT ELBOW

1.18 PRONATION, RIGHT ELBOW

elbows is to turn the hands up, as if carrying a bowl of soup (Figure 1.17); pronation is to turn the hands downward, like the hand position of Dandasana with the arms straight at your side, palms on the floor (Figure 1.18). Remember, these actions

are only done at the elbow joints and do not involve the shoulder joint.

At the ankles, supination is a position in which the sole of the foot is turned upward. This sometimes happens when you sit in Baddha Konasana.

A sudden extreme supination of the foot during weight bearing is what causes a sprained ankle. Pronation of the ankle is the opposite, a position in which the medial malleolus of the tibia moves distally, away from the knee joint, and the arch of the foot is pressed toward the floor.

Plantar flexion and dorsiflexion are other special movements. Plantar flexion is pointing the foot downward, like a ballerina's foot, so that the angle between the foot and the shin is increased (Figure 1.19); dorsiflexion is pulling the foot up toward the tibia, so the angle between the foot and tibia is decreased (Figure 1.20). Both of these movements occur at the ankle. Inversion of the foot is a combination of supination of the ankle and adduction of the forefoot; it is freer in plantar flexion. Eversion is pronation of the ankle in combination with adduction of the forefoot and is freer while the ankle is in dorsiflexion.

All movements occur in three planes: frontal, sagittal, and transverse. The frontal plane divides the body into anterior (front) and posterior (back). But it is also correct to use the words *anterior* and *posterior* as relative terms. For example, in the anatomical position, the hands are slightly anterior to the shoulder joints.

Movements in the frontal plane are the movements of abduction and adduction. These are movements parallel to the frontal plane and thus are said to be in the frontal plane. The arms in standing poses are moving in the frontal plane.

The next plane is the mid-sagittal, which divides the body into left and right sides and also is visualized along the midline, which runs between the eyes, through the sternum and navel, and down between the legs toward the feet.

Points that are closer to the midline are said to be medial, or proximal, while points that are farther from the midline are lateral or distal. For example, the shoulder joint is lateral to the nose; the navel is medial to the elbow. However, it is possible to refer to a medial point on the elbow, even though that structure itself is a lateral one in relationship to the elbow.

A parallel movement to the sagittal plane would be to take the upper extremities over the head, as in Vrksasana, also called flexion of the shoulder joint. Another movement in the sagittal plane is the position of the upper extremity in Urdhva Dhanurasana.

The third plane in which movement happens is the transverse plane, which divides the body in a plane parallel to the floor. If one starts from anatomical position, all rotation occurs in the transverse plane, whether it is the rotation of the vertebral column in a seated twist or the rotation of the

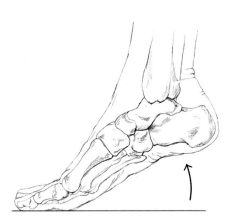

1.19 PLANTAR FLEXION, RIGHT ANKLE

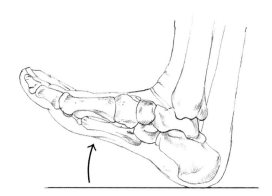

1.20 DORSIFLEXION, RIGHT ANKLE

arm at the straight elbow from the supination of the anatomical position to the opposite, pronation.

It is important to understand the planes of movement because of this fact: Muscles are more efficient when they contract in the plane in which they lie. For example, this means that because the triceps brachii lie in the sagittal plane, they are more efficient contracting in that plane. For an experiential understanding of this concept, see the next section.

Finally, there is a law of movement in joints, called the concave–convex law of joint movement, which can be helpful to understand and can be used to advantage when working with yoga students. It states that normal and maximal movement of a joint occurs when the concave surface of an articulation moves around the convex surface. What this means is that it is simply more effective when the concavity, or cave-like part of the joint, moves around the convex, or rounded end part of the joint.

To understand this law better, picture the hip joint. (While the hip joint is not a hinge joint, it is an easy example to picture when learning the concave–convex law.) In this example, the head of the femur is the convex surface, while the acetabulum, or hip socket, is the concave surface.

You move the femur in the acetabulum when you lie on your back and raise one leg up to perform Supta Padangusthasana or when bending forward in Uttanasana. Both are flexion of the hip joint, but only the second one follows the law, because in Uttanasana the concave acetabulum moves around and over the convex femoral head.

Many asana, including all the standing poses, follow the concave–convex law for the hip joint.

In Supta Padangusthasana, however, the opposite is true. Does this mean you should avoid poses like this that do not follow the law? Certainly not. It does mean, however, that if there is a problem with a certain joint or if someone is recovering from an injury, movements that follow the law will be more effective. We discuss this law in relationship to other joints as we move through the body.

EXPERIENTIAL ANATOMY

For Practicing

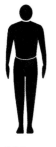

Applied Practice 1: Finding Your Own Bony Prominences
Prop: 1 nonskid mat
Take Care: These bony prominences are not covered by a lot of muscle or fat, so press gently to avoid creating soreness.
STAND IN TADASANA on your nonskid mat (Figure 1.21). Locate the following on your body: the lateral tip of the acromion, the coracoid process, the sternoclavicular joint, the greater trochanter of the femur, the medial and lateral malleoli, and the symphysis pubis.

1.21
TADASANA

Applied Practice 2: Experiencing Muscles Contracting In and Out of Their Planes in Chaturanga Dandasana
Prop: 1 nonskid mat
Take Care: Proceed gently if you have shoulder, elbow, or wrist problems.

GET DOWN on all fours on your nonskid mat. Place your hands under your shoulder joints and straighten the elbows. Reach back with each leg and, curling your toes, come onto the balls of your feet. Lower yourself into Chaturanga Dandasana, keeping your elbows close to your trunk (Figure 1.22). Notice the action of the triceps brachii, which are located in the back of your arms. Hold for a few breaths and release.

This is most efficient way of coming into Chaturanga Dandasana, because it uses the triceps in the sagittal plane, that is, the plane in which they lie. Now come back to your hands and knees and place your hands a little wider apart than the shoulders. Extend your legs behind you. As you descend with an exhalation, allow the elbows to move out at an approximate 45-degree angle to the body (Figure 1.23). If you experience discomfort in your wrists, come out of the pose and position your hands even farther apart and turn your fingers medially, or inward, a bit.

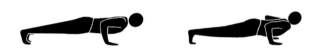

1.22 CHATURANGA DANDASANA, WITH THE ELBOWS CLOSE TO THE TRUNK

1.23 CHATURANGA DANDASANA, WITH THE ELBOWS OUT

This way of coming into Chaturanga Dandasana no longer places the triceps in the sagittal plane but in the frontal plane. Notice the difference from the first movement. You may find one easier and the other harder. If you find the second way easier, you may be stronger in the pectoral muscles of the upper and outer chest. They lie in the frontal plane and, with your elbows out to your side, the pectoral muscles can contract more efficiently, while the triceps cannot.

Push up into Chaturanga Dandasana with your hands and elbows in these two different positions and compare the difficulty of the movements.

For Teaching

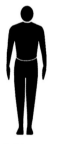

1.24
TADASANA

Applied Teaching 1: Finding the Bony Prominences on a Student or Teacher
Prop: 1 nonskid mat
Take Care: These bony prominences are not covered by a lot of muscle or fat, so press gently to prevent your student from becoming sore the next day.
WORK WITH A STUDENT or another yoga teacher to find these prominences on her body. I recommend that you ask for permission to touch her before beginning. Skip the symphysis pubis; just point it out to each other. Ask your student to stand in Tadasana on a nonskid mat (Figure 1.24). Locate the following: the lateral tip of the acromion, the corcoid process, the sternoclavicular joint, the spine of the scapula, the iliac crest, the sacroiliac joints, the greater trochanter, and the medial and lateral malleoli.

1.25
DANDASANA,
WITH ONE LEG
BENT AND THE
EXTENDED
ANKLE IN
DORSIFLEXION

Applied Teaching 2: Experiencing Accessory Joint Movement

Prop: 1 nonskid mat

Take care: Your student may feel very slight discomfort under the pressure of your hands but should not feel pain.

ASK YOUR STUDENT to sit in Dandasana on a nonskid mat, then bend both knees and put his feet on the floor. Have him straighten one leg and dorsiflex that ankle (Figure 1.25). Note the amount of movement on this side. Repeat on the other side as a compare.

Sit beside your student, facing in the same direction and slightly angled toward him. After asking permission to touch him, take hold of the anterior side of his right ankle with both hands, very firmly holding his lateral and medial malleolus together. Have him put his lower leg across your thigh so you can hold it easily. Ask him to dorsiflex his foot. He will not be able to do so or will only be able to do so a little. This is because you are preventing the accessory joint movement of the talus gliding.

What happens in normal dorsiflexion is that the distal tibia and fibula separate some to allow the talus to move slightly cranially and posteriorly. When you impede this separation of the distal fibula and tibia, dorsiflexion cannot occur. This is an example of the importance of accessory joint movement, in this case the slight separation of the distal tibia and fibula in dorsiflexion that occurs when walking.

LINK

To increase your powers of observation, whenever you can, spend some time observing the standing and walking postures of people in public places. You may find a lot of differences among cultures, ages, and genders. Note that how we stand and move is related to all these factors, as well as what work is being performed and what shoes are being worn.

The Muscles 2

YOU CAN DEVELOP GOOD JUDGMENT AS YOU DO THE MUSCLES OF YOUR BODY,
BY JUDICIOUS, DAILY EXERCISE. —GRANTLAND RICE

WE SPEND A lot of time in asana class stretching and strengthening muscles. While many students may not know much about their bodies when they begin the practice, they usually know the names of certain muscles, like the hamstrings, the biceps, and the abdominals. But as a yoga teacher, knowing where the muscles are, and how they work to create and shape actions, is a critical and useful skill. First, however, it helps to understand the relationship between muscles and bones.

BONES

Muscles are attached to bones at two locations; one is called the origin and the other the insertion (Figure 2.1). Muscles arise at the origin. This site is the more proximal of the two ends of the muscle and is considered to be the fixed end of attachment of the muscle during most movements. The muscle inserts at the distal end.

Muscles can originate and insert in the same region, like the muscles that start and stop on the hand. These are called intrinsic muscles. Extrinsic muscles arise in one region and pass to another, like the iliacus muscle, which originates on the pelvis and inserts on the femur.

However, origination and insertion can reverse, depending on the actions that are occurring. An example of the origin and insertion switching places can be seen with the latissimus dorsi muscle. It originates on the pelvis, on the connective tissue of the lumbar and sacral areas, on the thoracic and lumbar vertebrae, and on the lower ribs. It inserts on the intertubercular groove of the humerus, near the top medial portion of this bone, in the armpit area.

In most normal movements, the humerus is brought down toward the origin point, the pelvis, and other nearby areas. One example of this movement is swimming the butterfly stroke. The humerus, or insertion point, is brought toward the origin in the lower body.

However, when climbing a rope, the action is

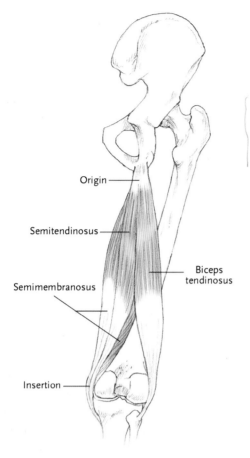

2.1 HAMSTRINGS: ORIGIN AND INSERTION
OF A TWO-JOINT MUSCLE

distal, this can vary, depending on what is stationary and what is moving at any given moment.

It is helpful to learn and remember as many origins and insertions as you can. Knowing where a muscle arises and where it ends will help you to understand not only the action that that muscle can make but also what might be going wrong if that muscle is not doing its job. Additionally, in order to stretch a muscle most effectively, knowing its attachments are critical. Take some time to memorize the origins and insertions of major muscles and their opposing muscles as they are specifically discussed in this book. Then use part of your of asana practice time to review and observe the origins and insertions in your own body. More details on the origins and insertions of individual muscles are presented in subsequent chapters.

JOINTS

Joints and muscles are intimately interactive. In fact a muscle can only act on a joint if it crosses that joint. For example, the brachio-radialis only crosses the elbow joint, so it can only act on the elbow joint. This type of muscle-joint relationship is the most common.

However, a muscle like as the biceps brachii of the humerus can act on more than one joint because it crosses two joints, in this case, the shoulder and elbow joints. This type of muscle is called a two-joint muscle. Some examples of two-joint muscles are the hamstrings, the quadriceps femoris (though only one head crosses two joints), and the biceps brachii (one head only). Since yoga practitioners are very familiar with the hamstrings, consider this example of how two-joint muscles work.

The hamstrings have four origins: three are on the ischial tuberositiy of the pelvis and one is on the linea aspera, the raised ridge on the posterior side of the femur. All of these heads of the hamstrings cross the knee, two inserting the knee at the medial tibia and two inserting at the lateral side of

reversed. The origin (lower body) is now brought upward toward the insertion (humerus) instead. To climb a rope, you fix, or stabilize, your arm and lift the pelvis toward the arms. Thus the origin and insertion points switch places in the action of rope climbing. Another movement that brings the insertion toward the origin occurs when pressing the humerus bones down while supporting your back with your hands in Salamba Sarvangasana. In this case, you fix the insertion, the humerus, and move the origin toward it to move your pelvis backward, to create the slight back bending movement needed to lift the chest in the pose.

Therefore it should be remembered that, while the origin and insertion are usually proximal and the knee. Because the hamstrings cross the hip joint and the knee joint, they can act on both joints and are two-joint muscles.

When the hamstrings contract, they extend the hip joint, bringing the femur backward from the anatomically neutral position. They flex the knee as well. The hamstrings can also help to rotate the tibia laterally or medially. The biceps femoris helps to rotate the tibia laterally after the knee joint is flexed. The semitendinosus and the semimembranosus help to rotate the tibia medially after the knee is flexed.

To feel these rotations, sit at the edge of a simple, straight chair, with your knees at an approximate angle of 90 degrees. Hold your distal femur so your hands make a circle around it, thumbs on top and the fingers to the back. You should be able to feel the hamstring tendons, especially on the medial side just proximal to the knee joint.

Now flex your hip joint about one-third of the way toward your chest and hold it there. Externally rotate your knee out to the side as for Padmasana. Notice the contraction under your fingers on the lateral hamstring tendons, the biceps femoris. Then reverse the rotation of the femur and tibia, as for going into Virasana. You will notice a contraction of the medial hamstrings, the semitendinosus, and the semimembranosus just above the medial knee joint, as they rotate the tibia.

Here is another suggestion that may help you understand the actions of the hamstrings better. Stand in Tadasana on a nonskid mat. Now move one leg backward (so you are standing only on one leg), and bend that knee so the heel of the foot lifts toward the ceiling. The position you are in is of being ready to kick a ball.

These two actions are largely created by the hamstring muscles. You can do these actions, extending the hip and flexing the knee, separately or together, but in either case these actions are mainly created by the hamstring muscles acting as two-joint muscles across two joints.

CONNECTIVE TISSUE

The fascial planes, or sheaths, are a network of connective tissue throughout the body that helps to hold it together and to maintain its shape. Specifically the connection of muscles to bones occurs through aggregates of connective tissue fibers known as tendons.

A tendon grows out of the bone matrix and periosteal covering of the bone, then becomes a connective tissue matrix that goes through and around the muscle, and then attaches at the other end to the bone by a tendon as well. Thus tendons are named for the muscle of which they are a part. Probably the best way to think of a tendon is as an extension or part of the muscle, not as a separate structure. Tendons, of course, do not have the same contractile elements as muscles.

Most muscles connect directly to the periosteum of the bone via tendons, but some muscles are attached to an aponeurosis. This is, in effect, a flattened tendon, a broad, flat, fibrous sheet of connective tissue that attaches to bone and to muscle. One example of an aponeurosis is the structure that the abdominal muscles attach onto at the anterior surface of the body.

MUSCLES

To understand how to stretch a muscle well, you must first know the origin and insertion points. Stretching a muscle happens by reversing the action or actions that it creates when contracting. Consider the abdominal muscles, which run all along the front of the body. When contracted, they approximate, or bring together, the rib cage and pelvis, such as when doing a sit-up. Therefore, to stretch the abdominals, it is necessary to perform the opposite of flexion, which is extension of the trunk. Back bends extend the trunk and therefore stretch the abdominal muscles.

In order to stretch effectively in the case of two-joint muscles, the stretch must be created over both joints simultaneously. For example, the hamstrings are hip extensors, and, to stretch them, hip flexion is needed. They are also knee flexors, so knee extension is needed as well. Thus an effective hamstring stretch is a position in which the hips are in flexion and the knees in extension, which happens in all forward bending asana.

The opposite of stretching a muscle is contracting it using metabolic energy. There are a number of specific characteristics of muscle contractions. One of these concerns contractibility and elasticity. Muscle fibers can contract to one-half of their resting length. They can also be stretched to half again as long as their resting length. Remember, muscles can contract, which requires metabolic work, and they can be stretched, but that is a passive process unless it is a lengthening contraction, such as in the example of lowering a book in your hand.

The second point to keep in mind when considering muscle contraction is the all-or-none law. This states that in each motor unit, other than in cardiac tissue, the individual muscle fiber is either contracting or not, just as a light switch is either on or off. Of course not all the motor units are involved each time you contract a muscle. The body uses only the number of units necessary to complete the movement. The harder the task, the more units are recruited. But each unit itself is either off or on.

The normal motor unit at rest is not firing at all. When measured on an electromyograph machine (EMG), there is no electrical potential or measurable charge in a muscle at rest. Interestingly enough, the concept of muscle tone is therefore not easily definable. Tone is not the state in which a muscle feels slightly contracted or firm to the touch, though we tend to use the word *tone* to mean this. One way to think of muscle tone is as the readiness to respond, but remember that at rest a normal muscle is not firing. Only a pathological muscle fiber fires at rest.

One of the most interesting characteristics of muscle contraction is that muscle motor units fire their fibers asynchronously. Keeping in mind the all-or-none law, imagine what would happen to your movement if groups of fibers or all the fibers fired together, all at once. If this happened, your movements would be jerky; each time you reached for something it would look like a car starting and stopping, as if the driver were pushing first the gas, then the brake, then the gas again. But the motor units do not fire this way. Because the motor units fire asynchronously, in more of an overlapping time sequence, the effect is that the movement is smooth. As some fibers stop firing, some are just starting, and vice versa, so that the movement is even.

Another characteristic of muscle firing is that a muscle contracts most efficiently when it contracts at a moderate speed. When it does so, its efficiency is approximately 20 to 25 percent, which is considered high compared to most machines. Quick movements are not as efficient, meaning that the extra energy needed for the quick movement is not proportionate to the speed gained. It is somewhat analogous to driving 55 mph; the higher your speed, the less efficiently the car burns fuel. Most asana are practiced at a moderate speed.

NERVES

A muscle receives its stimulation to contract from a motor nerve. The muscle and the nerve join at the neuromuscular junction (Figure 2.2). Each motor nerve branches to innervate many muscle fibers, but there is only one junction per muscle fiber. An electrical wave travels down the nerve fiber and is translated into a chemical reaction at the neuromuscular junction; this chemical energy travels across the gap between the nerve and muscle membranes. When the chemical transmitter reaches the muscle membrane, it is translated back into an electrical impulse that causes the muscle fiber to contract. The disease myasthenia gravis occurs when there is a chemical problem with the neurotransmitter found at the neuromuscular junction.

KINESIOLOGY

The single most important factor to understand when analyzing the movements created by muscles is the force of gravity. *All movements are shaped by the force of gravity.* Sometimes students of anatomy overlook this principle because it is so obvious.

Please recall the example in chapter 1 about coming down from Salamba Sirsasana (described on page 13). It was mentioned in the context of a lengthening contraction of the hamstrings. When your student comes out of Salamba Sirsasana, the force or power that creates the movement is gravity. There is no reason for the student to use any muscular effort to create the movement, because in this case gravity is the most efficient force to bring the legs down.

What the hamstring muscles are doing in this particular movement are acting as a brake to slow the descent of the legs toward the floor, thus protecting the muscles from too quick a descent. The hamstrings are not needed to act as creators of the movement, because gravity creates the movement with less metabolic energy expended by the body. The hamstrings only need to guide or shape the movement.

Another example of gravity creating a movement occurs during the practice of Uttanasana. Try this: stand on a nonskid mat, with your feet 12 inches apart, knees straight. On your next exhalation, bend forward to place your hands on the floor. As you do so, notice what is happening to your hamstrings, gluteus muscles, and erector spinae muscles. These muscles are not flexors of the hip, but extensors of your hip joint and vertebral column. Yet they act to create flexion of the hip by letting go with gravity to help control the downward movement. Gravity is already pulling

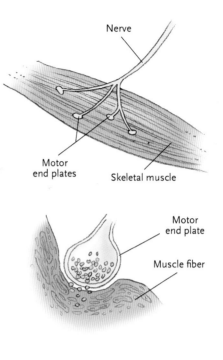

2.2 MUSCLE MOTOR UNIT

down on the trunk, and the extensors just need to slow down the movement, not create it. To use hip flexors to create Uttanasana would be redundant and would waste energy. Instead the body chooses to create the movement with the least energy necessary, a lengthening contraction of the hip extensors and erectors.

All joint movement either with or against gravity is synchronized through the interplay of three different functions that muscles can assume at different times. The first is when a muscle acts as the prime mover, or agonist. This is the term for whatever muscle creates the specific movement. An example of an agonist is the deltoid muscle in the upper outer arm initiating abduction of the humerus. Another example is the anterior tibialis of the lower anterior leg initiating the movement of dorsiflexion of the foot. Both of these muscles are originating the movement and thus are said to be agonists.

The second way a muscle can function is when

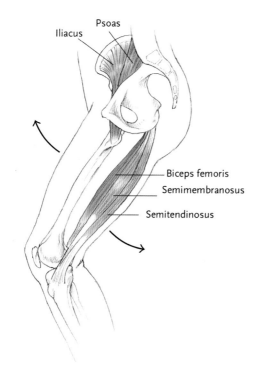

Iliacus
Psoas
Biceps femoris
Semimembranosus
Semitendinosus

2.3 HAMSTRINGS, AS ANTAGONISTS OF HIP FLEXORS
DURING RUNNING

it acts as the antagonist, in direct opposition to the agonist. The antagonist is the stabilizer of the movement. It acts as a brake on the movement. An example of a stabilizer, or antagonist, is the hamstring muscles when you run.

During the act of running, one of the agonists is the hip flexors, that is, the iliopsoas muscles. When they contract, they bring the femur forward into flexion; the hamstrings, which are hip extensors, contract to slow the powerful momentum of the swinging leg as it goes forward. In this case, the hamstrings are the antagonists (Figure 2.3). They help to shape or stabilize the positioning of the femur as it moves forward, to keep it from going too far. If the hamstrings did not slow down the strong forward movement of the femur during running, the femur would move forward into a high kick.

Agonists and antagonists act together in a very special way that is controlled by a principle called reciprocal innervation. Innervation is the stimulation of a muscle by a nerve. In this case, the principle states that as contraction occurs in an agonist, or prime mover, contractile activity diminishes at an equal rate it its antagonist. An example is the action of the muscles around the knee.

When the quadriceps femoris muscle contracts, it extends the knee joint. When the hamstrings at the back of the thigh contract, they help to flex the knee joint. If both muscles are contracting at the same time with the same force, no movement will be possible. This may be very desirable if one wants to hold a position, for example, a partially bent but stabilized knee in Virabhadrasana II. But in order for movement created by the agonist to occur, the antagonist must release at the same rate that the agonist contracts. This allows for smooth and efficient movements.

The third type of muscle function is slightly more complicated to understand. This is when a muscle acts as a neutralizer. A neutralizer is a muscle that prevents one of the actions of an agonist. A perfect example is the action of the adductors of the thigh during Urdhva Dhanurasana. In order to practice this pose, the extensors of the hip joint must all be contracting strongly to overcome the force of gravity and thus lift the body up. These extensors include the extensors of the vertebral column and the extensors of the hip joint, which are the hamstring muscles, the posterior gluteus medius, the gluteus maximus, with some help from the hip external rotators. The actions of the gluteus maximus are twofold: extension of the hip joint (as previously mentioned) and external rotation of the hip joint.

When practicing Urdhva Dhanurasana, many teachers instruct their students not to externally rotate the hip joints, thus separating and rolling out the thighs, yet is it common to see students doing it. This external rotation is evidenced by the student's feet turning out and the knees separating wider than the feet. When the femur externally rotates, this new relationship between the acetabulum and the femoral head interferes with the ability of the pelvis to move backward over the femoral head. The pelvis gets a bit stuck while trying to move backward when the femurs are in external rotation.

To feel this inhibition, stand on a nonskid mat with your feet 14 to 16 inches apart, turn your feet out, thus externally rotating the femurs, and move backward, as if you are going to drop back into a back bend. Note how your pelvis seems to get stuck in the process. Now try the same action with your feet turned inward; it will feel much easier and may relieve pressure or stress in your lower back as well.

Remember that the gluteus maximus does two things: extends the hip joint and externally rotates it. In Urdhva Dhanurasana, we want the hip extension aspect to lift the body from the floor. But most teachers do not want the external rotation aspect. What teachers often recommend is for the student to push the knees together, perhaps even adding a yoga block between the knees to press against.

This adduction movement of the thighs is created by the adductor muscles. The adductor muscles are the internal rotators of the hip joint, the opposite of the external rotators. Thus, by using the adductors in Urdhva Dhanurasana, the student is activating the adductors to act as a neutralizing agent against the external rotation component of the gluteus maximus muscle, while at the same time fully allowing the hip extension function.

EXPERIENTIAL ANATOMY

For Practicing

2.4
ANJANEYASANA, WITH BACK KNEE BENT

Applied Practice 1: Stretching Two-Joint Muscles

Props: 1 nonskid mat • a wall

Take Care: Balance can be a challenge, so use the wall if you need it.

PLACE THE SHORT END of your nonskid mat against the wall. Stand on the mat, facing the wall, and begin in Tadasana. For stability, you can place your left hand on the wall. Bend the right knee and catch your ankle with your hand, keeping your knees close together. Gently but firmly press your heel toward your buttock. This action will stretch the quadriceps femoris muscle over the knee joint. But because your hip is in neutral, you are not completely stretching the muscle. To do so, try the following pose.

Kneel on your mat and bring your right foot forward between your hands in Anjaneyasana (Figure 2.4). Keep your back leg straight at first, with your toes curled under, and press your pelvis down. Notice the stretch in the front of your back thigh. Now slowly begin to press your pelvis down, while slightly resisting from your back thigh. Lower your back thigh slowly but persistently. This will cause the quadriceps femoris to stretch, not only over the knee joint but also over the hip joint. The stretch will be more intense because it is over both joints of a two-joint muscle.

To continue the stretch, gradually bring your back knee to the floor, and then press forward a bit with your pelvis. You will feel even more stretch if you bring your back heel toward your buttock (as shown). If you try this movement, make sure you keep your pelvis down, and do not let it lift as the heel comes up.

Make sure that your knee remains directly over your front heel throughout all these variations to protect your knee joint from strain. Hold each variation for several breaths and then release. Now get up and walk around the room to notice the difference in how your leg and hip feel. Be sure to repeat to the other side.

Another way to experience the effect of stretching a two-joint muscle is to stretch the calf. Two big muscles make up most of the calf, the more superficial gastrocnemius and the deeper soleus. The gastrocnemius arises from the medial and lateral epicondyles of the femur and the posterior head and upper shaft of the fibula, while the soleus arises solely from the posterior tibia. Both muscles insert with a common tendon, the Achilles, which is attached to the calcaneus bone.

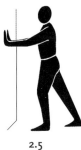

2.5

GASTROC-
NEMIUS
STRETCH,
AT THE WALL

To feel the difference between stretching the soleus, a one-joint muscle, and the gastrocnemius, a two-joint muscle, try the following. Face the wall and stand in Tadasana on your nonskid mat, and place your hands at shoulder level. Now step your right foot back about 12 to 18 inches. Make sure that your foot is straight, so the outside of your foot is parallel to the edge of your mat. Now lean forward by bending your left knee, while keeping your back heel firmly on the floor (Figure 2.5). You may need to adjust the position of your back foot by moving it backward or forward a bit. Continue to be meticulous about not turning your heel inward. This pose will stretch the gastrocnemius muscle across both joints, the knee and the ankle.

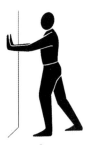

2.6

SOLEUS
STRETCH,
AT THE WALL

Now bend your back knee directly over the forefoot, without lifting your heel. This movement takes out the stretch of the gastrocnemius across the knee joint by releasing the stretch at that end of the muscle, thus focusing the stretch on the other end of the joint and on the soleus muscle (Figure 2.6). You will probably feel the stretch just from the mid-calf downward in the soleus as well as in the Achilles tendon. Throughout this stretch, remember to keep your breathing relaxed and natural. After stretching on one side, be sure to repeat on your left side.

Applied Practice 2: Focusing on Stabilization
Prop: 1 nonskid mat
Take Care: Lie in a symmetrical position. Do not lie on your back if you are more than four months pregnant.
LIE DOWN on your back on your nonskid mat as for Savasana, with your feet comfortably apart and your arms away from your torso, palms up (Figure 2.7). Close your eyes and

2.7
SAVASANA

relax for several cycles of breath. When you feel relaxed, try this experiment. First simply imagine that you are going to lift your straight right leg. Pay exquisite attention to what is happening in your body as you think the movement before actually performing it.

The very first thing you will probably notice is your left abdominal muscles contracting.

Very quickly you will probably begin to feel other muscles contracting, for example, your left gluteus maximus, left hamstrings, lower back muscles, even your shoulder muscles. Notice how you gradually recruit more and more muscles. The stronger the action (that is, the higher you lift your leg) either in reality or in your imagination, the more muscles are needed to stabilize the desired motion

For Teaching

2.8
UTTANASANA

Applied Teaching 1: Isolating the Hamstrings as a Limitation to Forward Bends
Prop: 1 nonskid mat
Take Care: Avoid this if your student is uncomfortable bearing weight on her knees.
MANY YOGA STUDENTS have problems bending forward because of tight hamstring muscles, and yoga teachers are often concerned with how to help them. First have the student stand on a nonskid mat and come into Uttanasna (Figure 2.8). Notice how her pelvis is tilting forward to create the forward bend. Is her back rounded, or is her sacrum tilting down? Remember, the healthiest forward bends for the lower back are done with the pelvis tilting. The more the sacrum tilts, the more the hamstrings have to lengthen, and the more the action is created through the hip joints and not by the more delicate lower back flexing too much, thus putting pressure on the intervertebral discs.

Now, to ascertain whether the student's difficulty is the direct result of tight hamstrings or instead a problem with her hip joints or lower back, try the following. Have her kneel down on all fours on a nonskid mat. Then ask her to move her tailbone down, which will create lumbar flexion, and then tailbone up, which will create lumbar extension (Figures 2.9 and 2.10). Her pelvis will very likely move quite freely up and down over the hip joints, even if she has tight hamstrings.

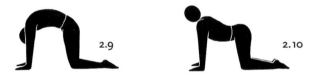

2.9

2.10

2.9
ALL FOURS,
TAILBONE
DOWN

2.10
ALL FOURS,
TAILBONE UP

By placing her in the bent-knee position, you have eliminated the stretch of the hamstrings over the knee joint. Most students will find the tipping of the pelvis, which they found difficult in a standing forward bend, much easier to do on all fours.

If trying this movement on all fours has not improved her ability to move the pelvis, there is very likely some problem other than tight hamstrings, possibly a problem with her hip joint(s), and I would suggest she get a diagnosis from a health care professional trained in orthopedics. Once the student has experienced the ease of tipping her pelvis in a forward bend–like movement on her hands and knees on the floor, she will have a better idea of how to do it in Uttanasana. And as her teacher, you will have more confidence that her hips and back are healthy.

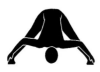

2.11

PRASARITA
PADOTTAN-
ASANA

Applied Teaching 2: Making Hamstring Stretching Easier

Prop: 1 nonskid mat

Take Care: Make sure the student does not experience any lower back pain during this practice.

HELPING STUDENTS bend forward more easily is related to how far apart the legs are. When the legs are close together, the hamstrings are stretched directly in a straight line from hip joints to knees. When the student widens his legs in a pose such as Prasarita Padottanasana, the hamstrings are no longer in a straight line, and the stretch on them is less direct (Figure 2.11). The student will no doubt feel less stretch on the hamstrings in this position, and if hamstrings are his primary limitation, he will find Prasarita Padotta-nasana a much easier pose to practice.

LINK

To continue an in-depth study of the muscles and their actions, I recommend *Muscles: Testing and Function, 4th ed.,* by Florence Peterson Kendall and Elizabeth Kendall McCreary (Philadelphia: Lippincott Williams & Wilkins, 1993).

PART TWO:

The Vertebral Column

Introduction to the Vertebral Column 3

GOOD HEALTH COMES FROM A STRAIGHT SPINE AND A CLEAN COLON.

—HINDU PROVERB

DURING MY TRAINING to become a physical therapist, I spent a lot of time studying the spinal column, its bones, its nerves, and the kinesiological functions of this part of the body. In the evenings after classes, a group of us would sometimes stay a little late to avoid the evening traffic jam on the bridge and would spend our time studying together in a relaxed manner. One of the things we would do was to pick up an individual vertebra from a box we had in our lab and, without looking at it, attempt to identify not only the region of the spine it came from but which bone it was. We got pretty good at this game. While yoga teachers may not need this level of expertise, knowing as much as you can about the vertebral column and its functions will be of great help in your teaching.

Most asana are concerned with maintaining the health and movement of the spinal column. It is generally accepted by most teachers that the spine is not only at the core of our structure but also at the core of our practice. However, what surprises most teachers as they begin to study this part of the body in depth is how distinct each section, even each vertebrae, is one from the other. This section of *Yogabody* begins with an overview chapter on the column as a whole and then offers a chapter on each region of the spinal column.

BONES

The vertebral column, also called the spinal column, consists of thirty-three bones, not all of which are independently movable. Contrary to the proverb at the beginning of this chapter, the bones of the column are arranged in a series of gentle curves from top to bottom. These curves can best be seen from the sagittal, or side, view (Figure 3.1).

There are five sections of the column. The most superior is the cervical region, or neck, and consists of seven vertebrae. They are numbered, as are all vertebrae, from the top down. The next region is the thoracic spine, with twelve vertebrae; all thoracic vertebrae are attached to two ribs each. The lumbar spine and the sacrum each consist of five vertebrae, except the sacrum's are fused into one curved bone. The coccyx is made up of three to five vertebrae and is commonly called the tailbone.

The vertebrae are named for their region, using the first letter of the region and numbered from the top down, like this: C1, T8, L4. These vertebrae would be the first cervical, eighth thoracic, and fourth lumbar, respectively.

The vertebral column has a variety of functions, including helping to holding us upright and providing an armature for the posterior wall of the trunk and ribs. Additionally these bones protect the nerves of the spinal cord and serve as the attachment site of muscles and ribs, thus helping to protect the internal organs.

The spinal column plays a major part in all of our movements, especially in the movements of asana. In yoga there are philosophical implications to the vertebral column as well as the more obvious anatomical and kinesiological ones. The spiritual energy of *kundalini* is said to lie curled like a sleeping serpent at the base of the spine. It is the awakening of this energy, as it travels upward along the *sushumna*, an esoteric canal at the center of the spinal column, until it reaches the highest center in the brain. When this happens, it is believed that the practitioner has attained the state of enlightenment.

However, from a structural viewpoint, the most significantly observable aspect of the column is that it is arranged in a series of curves, which can be easily viewed from the side, and is not a straight line. This series of curves allows for freer movement between the segments and improves the ability of the column to bear weight efficiently and act as a shock absorber. The vertebral curves are called "normal curves" by anatomists, thus underscoring their importance.

The thoracic spine at the rib cage area and the sacral curve below the waist are called primary curves because they are developed in utero. These two regions of the spinal column remain curved in the same direction throughout life. Both of these curves have their concavity anteriorly. Because the thoracic and sacral spines have their concavity anteriorly, they are said to exhibit a kyphosis. The word *kyphosis* refers to the curve itself; in the common vernacular, however, the word *kyphotic* is often used to mean too much of this type of curve.

The cervical curve and the lumbar curve are both called secondary curves because they develop after birth. These curves have their concavity posteriorly and are said to be lordotic. The term *lordotic* is often used to mean too much of a lordosis in one of these curves.

In utero the baby is in flexion, the direction of the primary (thoracic and sacral) curves. As the baby begins to hold her head up, the cervical curve develops; her lumbar curve develops while she is learning to stand. Because the secondary curves are developed and are the opposite of the curve of the column found in utero, they are less stable. It is much more common for yoga students to have problems with either the cervical or lumbar region than the thoracic or sacral, in part because of this lessened stability.

The secondary curves are said to be sympathetic curves. This means that when your student flexes his neck, he also has a tendency to flex his lumbar spine, and when he extends his lumbar spine, he often will extend his cervical spine as well. You can experiment with this. Lie on your back, knees bent, on your nonskid mat. Close your eyes and take a few easy breaths to relax and center. Now draw your lower back toward the floor, and notice your neck: it also flattens and lowers toward the floor. Extend your cervical spine by lifting your chin and increasing the curve, and notice what happens to your lumbar spine: it also extends and moves away from the floor. Remember the concept

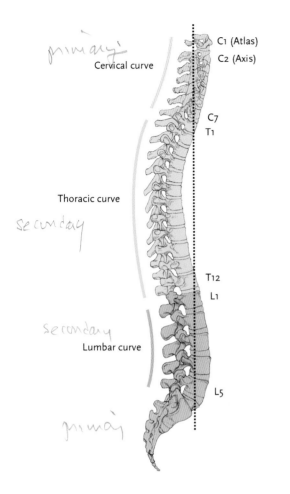

primary

Cervical curve

C1 (Atlas)
C2 (Axis)

C7
T1

Thoracic curve

secondary

T12
L1

secondary

Lumbar curve

L5

primary

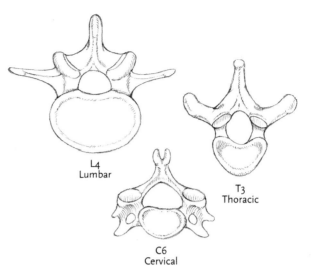

L4
Lumbar

T3
Thoracic

C6
Cervical

3.1 (LEFT) NORMAL CURVES OF THE VERTEBRAL COLUMN, WITH SAGITTAL VIEW OF PLUMB LINE

3.2 (ABOVE) CERVICAL, THORACIC, AND LUMBAR VERTEBRAE, SHOWING THE SHAPE OF THE BODY; SUPERIOR VIEW)

of sympathetic curves when you are teaching forward bends and back bends.

Each vertebra has a body, which is the largest single portion of the vertebra. The exceptions are C1 and C2. C1 lacks a body entirely, and C2 has a small, roundish body. When viewed superiorly or inferiorly, the vertebral bodies have a different shape in each vertebral region. In the cervical region, the bodies are oblong; the thoracic bodies have a heart-shaped form; and the lumbar bodies appear kidney-shaped (Figure 3.2).

The body is the main weight-bearing part of the vertebra. Note that the vertebral bodies increase in size, from cervical to lumbar, in order to better support the weight from above. The ends of each vertebral body are covered superiorly and

inferiorly with a cartilage end plate. There is also an opening in the body to allow for nourishment from the blood supply. Remember, bones are living tissue and, as such, need oxygen and other nourishment.

C1, which does not have a body, is instead shaped like an oval or oblong ring. Embryologists tell us that the body of C1 migrates distally during embryological development and fuses with C2 to create a prominence on the anterior body of C2 called the dens, or odontoid process. The second cervical vertebra can then rotate on C1 around the dens.

The vertebral arch is the bony ring in the middle of each vertebral body and is the opening for the passage of the spinal cord. Note that the cord is located at the most protected part of the column. The anterior part of this circular structure, which connects to the body, is called the pedicle; the posterior portion of the arch is called the lamina.

From the lateral view, the inferior and superior vertebral notches, or bony arches, are apparent. The vertebral notch creates part of the opening for the spinal nerve to pass out laterally from the cord. There is a superior and an inferior vertebral notch. The vertebral notch from one vertebra fits together with the vertebral notch of the one below it. This is like placing the two halves of a doughnut together to make a circle. The circle it creates is called the vertebral foramen, or opening, through which the root of the spinal nerve of the spinal cord passes. Actually the spinal nerve root only takes up two-thirds of the total space in the vertebral foramen. The rest of the space is taken up by a protective envelope around the nerve root. This envelope consists of fatty tissue, loose connective tissue, and blood and lymph vessels.

The lateral transverse processes, or bony projections, are found on the lateral sides of the vertebrae. The transverse bony processes emerge between the pedicle and the lamina. These processes serve as the attachment points for muscles. Think of a transverse process like the handlebars of a bicycle. When you turn your handlebars to the right, the front wheel turns right. The opposite occurs, of course, when you turn left. The transverse processes of the vertebral column function similarly. When muscles on one side of the transverse process contract, they help to rotate the vertebral body.

The other process on the vertebral body points posteriorly; it is called the spinal process, and it emerges from the lamina. The spinal process is the knobby protuberance you can feel and sometimes see down the central "canal" of the column when you look at your student's back. The spinal process serves as the attachment point for ligaments and muscles. It can be easily palpated. Try this.

Have your student get on all fours on his non-skid mat. As he exhales, have him lift and round his vertebral column. After asking permission to touch, run your fingers along his spine, feeling the pointed spinous processes. You may note that some are more prominent than others or that the spaces between them are slightly irregular. Or you may find that some seem rotated to one side.

Yoga teachers often express concern that the prominence of these spinal processes in forward bends is incorrect. This may not be totally appropriate. Some students may have more of a lumbar curve, so the processes are not as easily seen or felt. Others may have longer spinal processes, so that the processes are more prominent. It is more important to take into account the entire shape of the column and the positioning of the pelvis when accessing the health of a forward bend, not just the appearance of the spinal processes.

Joints

Each vertebral body has four flattened surfaces, called facets, on the posterior side, which are covered with cartilage to facilitate fluid movement and to protect the bony surfaces. Two face upward, the superior facet surfaces, and two face downward, the inferior facet surfaces. These are the sites where adjacent vertebrae meet to form a joint, the face joint. However, the sacrum only has two superior facet joints, and they join superiorly with L5.

The facet joints lie at different angles in each of the movable sections of the column. In the cervical region, the superior facets are at an angle of approximately 45 degrees, facing posteriorly and upward (Figure 3.3). The superior thoracic facets face backward but are more vertical than the cervical facets (Figure 3.4). The superior lumbar facets face medially, except the L5-S1, which face almost posteriorly (Figure 3.5). The change from cervical to thoracic facet angles is gradual, but the change from thoracic to lumbar facet angles is abrupt.

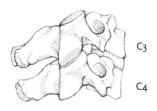

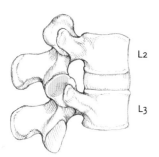

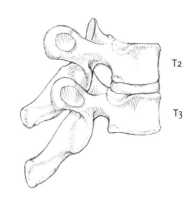

C3

C4

T2

T3

L2

L3

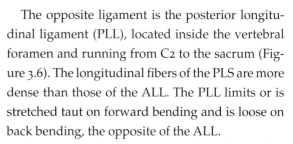

Occipital protuberance

Ligamentum nuchae

C7

Supraspinal ligament

Interspinal ligaments

Anterior longitudinal ligament

Posterior longitudinal ligament

3.3 (TOP LEFT) CERVICAL FACET JOINT ANGLE

3.4 (TOP MIDDLE) THORACIC FACET JOINT ANGLE

3.5 (ABOVE LEFT) LUMBAR FACET JOINT ANGLE

3.6 (RIGHT) ANTERIOR LONGITUDINAL LIGAMENT AND POSTERIOR LONGITUDINAL LIGAMENT, INCLUDING UNIQUE L5 AND S1 AREAS

(The unique features of the facet joints at the transitional segments—C7-T1, T12-L1, and L5-S1—are discussed in the individual chapters about these regions.)

CONNECTIVE TISSUE

The bodies of the vertebrae are held together by two ligaments and the intervertebral discs. The anterior longitudinal ligament (ALL) is a very strong ligament located on the anterior surface of the bodies of the vertebrae from C2 to the sacrum (Figure 3.6). In fact some consider it the strongest ligament in the body. It is thickest in the thoracic region. It prevents the vertebrae from moving forward. The ALL is stretched in back bending and loosened in forward bending.

The opposite ligament is the posterior longitudinal ligament (PLL), located inside the vertebral foramen and running from C2 to the sacrum (Figure 3.6). The longitudinal fibers of the PLS are more dense than those of the ALL. The PLL limits or is stretched taut on forward bending and is loose on back bending, the opposite of the ALL.

The bodies of the vertebrae are also held together by a special kind of connective tissue known as the intervertebral discs. In fact the twenty-three discs are the main connectors between the bodies of the vertebrae. There is no disc between the skull and C1 or between C1 and C2.

The disc is the most important structure for the preservation of the function of the vertebral column. A healthy and plump disc helps maintain the range of motion (ROM) at the adjacent vertebral segment. Plump discs also help to keep the bodies of the vertebrae an appropriate distance apart. This helps to maintain the space necessary to prevent any impingement on the spinal nerve from the vertebral body. When the disc is compressed, it allows the vertebrae to approximate, and this can contribute to pressure on a spinal nerve.

Discs are unique in each region of the column. The cervical discs are thicker anteriorly and are smaller than their cervical bodies. The thoracic discs have the same anterior to posterior measurements as the body but are more narrow. This particular structure contributes to the relative restriction of the upper thoracic compared to the lower thoracic spine. The lumbar discs are higher anteriorly, particularly L5, which contributes to the creation of the lumbo-sacral angle. In the lower lumbar, the lordosis is formed by the discs and by the shape of the bodies, while in the upper lumbar, the curve is due to the discs entirely.

The cartilage that covers the ends of the vertebral bodies is called the cartilage endplate. The endplates of two adjacent vertebral bodies are connected by fifteen to eighteen layers of fibers called Sharpes ligaments. The outer layers are more vertical, while the innermost layers are more horizontal. This layered structure increases the stability of the connection.

Whenever you rotate the column, these endplates approximate, or move together, thus compressing the intervertebral disc. A simple example of how this works is to observe what happens when you wring and twist a towel to remove excess water. As your turn the towel, your hands come closer together. This is basically what happens to the layers of the disc whenever you perform a twisting asana. Even though we suggest to our students the image of lengthening during twisting, an image I find helpful, it is important to remember that what is actually happening is that the vertebral bodies are approximating, and the discs are being compressed.

In the body, the discs are partially supported by the pressure created by the abdominal muscles and organs; this pressure helps to keep the discs in place.

Figure 3.7 shows the effects of movement on the discs. When you bend backward, the discs are pushed slightly forward. There is usually no problem with this movement, as it is away from the spinal nerve. The opposite is true in forward bending: when you flex the column, as in Paschimottanasana, your discs are pushed backward, in the direction of the spinal nerve. Thus forward bends and twists that compress the discs are not recommended for students suffering from an impingement of a spinal nerve. Besides the spinal nerve, the other painful structures in the vertebral column are the PLL and the facet joint.

The disc itself consists of circular ligaments called the annulus fibrosus. These circular rings are connected to the Sharpes ligaments. The center of the disc is composed of the nucleus pulposus, a semigelatinous substance that is the weight-bearing axis for all spinal movements. The nucleus pulposus has no direct blood supply after the third decade of life. Yet it is made up of 80 percent water. So what keeps the disc plump and full of water? Movement does it, by a process called imbibition.

Imbibition, from the verb "to imbibe or to drink," is the word used to describe the action of the disc passively taking up fluid from the surrounding tissue. Movement is what causes the disc to take up fluids. By bending forward, bending backward, and twisting, pressure on one side of the disc causes the other side of the disc to take up fluids passively, which helps it stay plump and healthy. When you bend forward, the back part of the disc is opened and can take in fluids; when you bend backward, the opposite happens. When we are young, the nucleus is full and contacts both cartilage endplates. As we age, the disc dries out, and this can lead to problems. Asana is an effec-

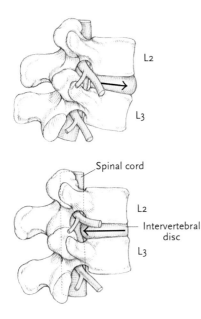

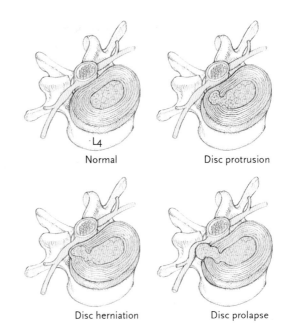

3.7 EFFECTS ON THE DISCS IN (TOP) BACK BENDING AND (BOTTOM) FORWARD BENDING

3.8 DISC PROTRUSION, DISC HERNIATION, AND DISC PROLAPSE OF THE NUCLEUS

tive way to move the column safely in all directions, thus helping to maintain the plumpness of the disc.

Figure 3.8 illustrates disc protrusion, disc herniation, and disc prolapse of the nucleus. The first sign of problems with discs is called protrusion. In this case, the nucleus moves out of its center location into the annulus. At this point, the student will not feel any numbness or tingling but may feel a deep, dull ache. Protrusion tends to happen in active people between the ages of twenty-five and forty. Herniation is the pathology in which the nucleus pushes against the edge of the annulus. The student may have as many as twenty attacks over time. True prolapse of the nucleus occurs when the nucleus moves outside the outer rim of the annulus and presses on the spinal nerve. This usually occurs with a movement that combines flexion and rotation and causes a sharp pain, which subsides. At that point, the student requires care from a health professional who specializes in the

care of ruptured discs. Bed rest or surgery may be required to alleviate the pain.

Yoga teachers should be very careful when a student experiences lower back pain; if the student complains of numbness, tingling, or radiating pain, or has problems with bowel and bladder control, send the person immediately to a health care professional. Yoga postures can be begun very slowly once the numbness becomes pain, as this means the nerve pressure is decreasing. Only very experienced teachers should attempt to work with these students.

The classic presentation of someone with a prolapsed disc is to stand with a deviation of the column to avoid the pain. If a student is deviating left to avoid right pain, for example, this means that the prolapse is lateral. If a student is deviating over the painful side, in this case deviating right over a right-sided lesion, then the prolapse is medial. This means that the prolapse is in the direction of the spinal cord, and very great care should be taken.

Usually an anterior prolapse causes much less pain and problem because it is into the ALL, which is not particularly painful. The three structures in the vertebral column itself are the PLL, the facet joints, and the nerve roots.

Another cause of radiating pain is when the piriformis muscle in the hip, one of the rotators, presses on the sciatic nerve as it exits the pelvis. Look for more discussion of this in chapter 8.

Here is an example of amount of pressure on the L3–L4 disc of a 154-pound man:

▶ lying on back: 66 pounds

▶ standing: 154 pounds

▶ upright sitting without support: 220 pounds

▶ sitting and bending forward 20 degrees: 264 pounds

▶ bent-knee sit-up: 396 pounds

▶ lifting a 44-pound weight with lumbar in flexion and knees straight: 748 pounds

Note: Thirty percent of weight in all positions (except lying) is dissipated by the muscles of the thorax and abdomen.

There are five ligaments that join other structures of the vertebral column together, other than the bodies:

▶ the ligamentum flavum (*flavum* means "yellow"), and it joins adjacent laminae from C2 to the sacrum. It is stretched in forward bending and twisting. It is loose on back bending. It also helps the spine return from flexion. It exerts a constant pull on the capsule of the lumbar facet joints to prevent the capsule from being caught in the facet joint upon movement.

▶ the supraspinal ligament attaches the points of the spinous processes from C7 to the sacrum. It is stretched on forward bending and twists and slack on back bending (Figure 3.9).

▶ the ligamentum nuchae is the portion of the supraspinal ligament that runs from the occipital protuberance to the spinal process of C7. It is stretched on flexion, as in dropping the head for chin lock and in Salamba Sarvangasana and Halasana.

▶ the interspinal ligaments connect adjoining spinous processes and run more along the side of these processes, connecting one process to the next. They are stretched on both twists and forward bends.

▶ the intertransverse ligaments run between the transverse processes. These ligaments are stretched in twisting poses.

Nerves

The spinal cord is the neural extension of the medulla oblongata of the brain. It exits the skull through the foramen magnum, or great opening. As a baby develops inside its mother, the spinal cord fills all the vertebral foramen from C1 to L5. But as the vertebral column continues to grow, the cord does not, so in the adult the cord ends at the distal end of the L2 vertebrae. At the end of the spinal cord, the nerves branch into the cauda equina, or horse's tail (Figure 3.10). This structure fills the lower vertebral canal.

There is a covering to the spinal cord called the meninges. This covering is divided into three layers: the outer is the toughest and thus is called the dura mater, which also forms a covering for the spinal cord, nerves, and the brain. The middle layer of the meninges is the arachnoid mater, so named because it resembles the filaments of a spider web. This layer gives some support to the spinal cord. Between the dura and arachnoid layers is the subdural space. The innermost layer adjacent to the spinal cord is the thin vascular pia mater, which is actually the outer layer of the spinal cord. The space between the arachnoid and pia mater is

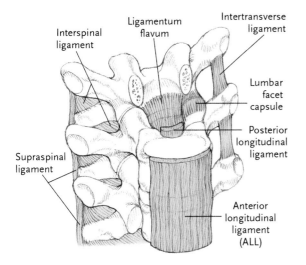

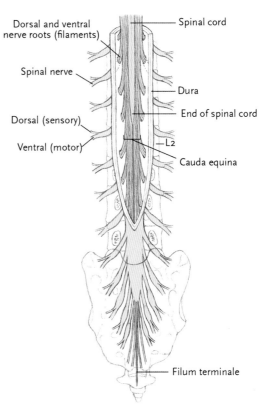

3.9 LIGAMENT NUCHAE, SUPRASPINAL LIGAMENT, AND LIGAMENTUM FLAVA (ABOVE)

3.10 CAUDA EQUINA (RIGHT)

called the subarachnoid space; it contains cerebrospinal fluid, which cushions the brain and spinal cord.

Nerves emerge on both sides, all along the spinal cord. The first spinal nerve exits between the skull and C1, the second spinal nerve exits between C1 and C2, and so forth. This means that there are eight spinal nerves but only seven vertebrae. The nerves, like the vertebrae, are numbered from the top down. So spinal nerve C4 exits the cord between C3 and C4. Then, beginning in the thoracic region, the nerves are named for the vertebral body just above them.

The spinal nerves have two divisions, the anterior and posterior roots. Each spinal nerve controls a certain part of the body (Figure 3.11). The anterior nerve root, sometimes called the ventral nerve root, controls the muscles as well as the glands and organs of that particular region. The posterior nerve root relays sensation, including pain, temperature, pressure, touch, and proprioception.

(*Proprioception* is "position sense," that is, the sense of knowing where your body is in space.) The area of the body controlled by one posterior, or dorsal, nerve root is called a dermatome (Figure 3.12). This is important to know because when the student complains of radiating pain, you will be able to make an educated guess if perhaps a nerve root is compressed and about which spinal nerve root might be involved.

The symptoms of nerve compression are tingling, pain, and numbness. The student may complain of these feelings in the arms down to the fingers or in the buttocks down to the feet. The farther the symptom is felt from the spinal nerve root, the more severe the nerve compression. Contrary to what may seem obvious, numbness is the worse sign. The job of the nerve is to carry impulses. When a person feels tingling, some pressure is beginning to interfere with the oxygen supply to the nerve; if this continues, the person will feel pain. If the compression continues, the person will then feel numb-

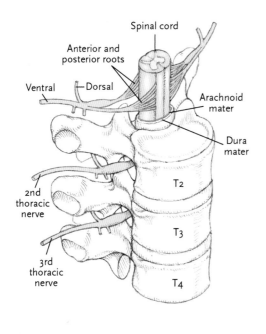

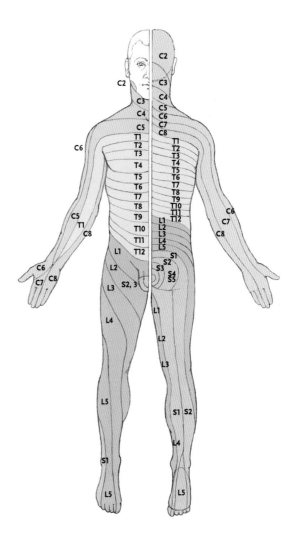

3.11 (ABOVE) SPINAL NERVE

3.12 (RIGHT) DERMATOMES

ness. When the compression is relieved, the sensation will go from numbness to pain to tingling to no abnormal sensation. Thus pain is a better symptom than numbness and means that the compression is beginning to be relieved.

Perhaps you can remember the feeling of sitting on your foot and it going to sleep. First it tingles, then it hurts, then it feels numb. When it wakes up, first it hurts, then it tingles, then it feels normal. This is a sign that the nerve is now receiving the appropriate amount of oxygen. Remember, nerves have a very high metabolic rate that requires a continual oxygen (O_2) supply, and they are exquisitely sensitive to the loss of it.

An example of temporary nerve compression is sometimes experienced by people with bulky and strong arms when they practice Salamba Sarvangasana, with their hands supporting the back. Students may complain of tingling, pins and needles, or even numbness in the hands. These symptoms could be occurring because the student is compressing the brachial nerves in the armpit as they exit the thorax. This is likely due to the tightness of the shoulder muscles.

If this occurs, recognize it as a neurological sign, a sign that a nerve is not receiving sufficient oxygen. Consider too that the nerve compression could be created in the cervical spine itself, by a disc pressing on the spinal nerve, or it could be created by compression on the nerve at any place along its path. My suggestion is that you assume the least problematic explanation for this condition, that is, that the compression is occurring somewhere else other than at the spinal nerve. However, if the problem persists, the student should consult a health practitioner.

To help your student, have him move his blanket setup to the wall and come up in Salamba Sarvangasana again, placing his hands on his back and keeping his feet on the wall for support. If the tingling returns, have him place his arms out to the side, so his armpits are totally open. In most cases the tingling will go away. This is because the nerves to the upper extremity pass through the armpit area on their way to innervate the upper extremities. When the student with tight or bulky shoulders presses his hands to the back, he can be compressing the nerves in his armpit and thus causing the tingling sensation. If taking his hands away from his back does not immediately give relief, ask the student to come out of the pose and refer him to a qualified health care professional for evaluation.

Muscles

There are numerous muscles on the posterior trunk. Many are muscles that connect the trunk to the upper extremity or muscles that connect the trunk to the pelvis. These muscles are discussed in the chapters 11 and 12.

At present, however, we will discuss the main extensor muscles specifically. These spinal muscles are a complicated overlapping group of muscles that act like a single muscle functionally to extend the column. We tend to refer to all the muscles that extend the column as the erector spinae. Technically, the erectors are only one of the three main parts of the muscles that extend the spinal column. The best way to understand these muscles is to study the illustrations (Figures 3.13, 3.15, and 3.17) and the charts (Figures 3.14, 3.16, and 3.18).

The intermediate layer of the extensor muscles of the back are the erector spinae muscles proper. They are a series of long muscles, lying medially to laterally, with overlapping origins and insertions. When they contract, they act as a group to extend the vertebral column. These muscles lie in the groove on the side of the vertebral column.

The iliocostalis, with thoracic and lumbar sections, is the most lateral of these muscles; the longissimus, with sections attaching to the skull, the cervical spine, and the thoracic spine, is slightly more medial. Finally, the spinalis, with a portion joining the skull, one joining in the cervical region, and one joining in the thoracic region, is the most medial. The semispinalis capitas is the final member of this group.

The deep layer of the extensor muscles of the back are the paravertebral transversospinalis, or the oblique group. Generally these muscles run from one transverse process to the spinous process of the vertebra above and span one to three vertebrae.

Kinesiology

The vertebral column can be thought of as a connected chain of moving parts, what kinesiologists call a kinetic chain. One way to visualize this is to think of the facet joints of each side of the column as a little column of its own. This column of facet joints moves as a whole. When one section becomes hypomobile, another section becomes hypermobile to take up the slack of the segment that is not moving well.

Each segment of the spine has a certain rhythm of movement. Try this with your student. Ask her to get on hands and knees on a nonskid mat. Have her begin to move her spinal column upward into flexion by beginning at the base of the skull so her head drops, then vertebra by vertebra, lifting each spinous process one by one. Suggest that she lift each vertebra one by one in the thoracic area as well, and then finally in the lumbar area. Repeat

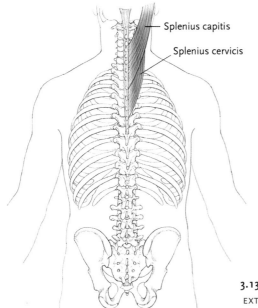

Splenius capitis

Splenius cervicis

3.13 SUPERFICIAL LAYER OF THE
EXTENSOR MUSCLES OF THE BACK

3.14 SUPERFICIAL LAYER OF THE EXTENSOR MUSCLES OF THE BACK

MUSCLE	ORIGIN	INSERTION	ACTION
Splenius capitis	Ligamentum nuchae and spinous processes of C6 and C7 vertebrae	Mastoid process and lateral ⅓ of ligamentum nuchae	Together with the splenius cervicis, extends the head and neck, unilaterally bends head and neck to side of contraction
Splenius cervicis	Ligamentum nuchae and spinous processes of C6 and C7 vertebrae	Posterior transverse processes of C1–C3 vertebrae	Together with the splenius capitis, extends head and neck, unilaterally bends head and neck to side of contraction

3.16   Intermediate Layer of the Extensor Muscles of the Back

Muscle	Origin	Insertion	Action
Iliocostalis: located most lateral to the vertebrae	Broad tendon from posterior sacrum, posterior iliac crest, sacral and lumbar spinous processes, and supraspinous ligament	Angles of lower ribs and cervical transverse processes	Together with left and right sides or with other erectors on both sides of column, extends vertebral column and head; unilaterally side bends vertebral column
Longissimus: located lateral to the spinalis	By broad tendon to posterior iliac crest, posterior sacrum, sacral and lumbar spinous processes, supraspinous ligament	Ribs and transverse processes of cervical and thoracic vertebrae; mastoid process of temporal bones	Together with left and right sides or with other erectors on both sides of column, extends vertebral column and head; unilaterally side bends vertebral column
Spinalis: located most medial to the vertebrae	By broad tendon to posterior iliac crest, posterior sacrum, sacral and lumbar spinous processes, supraspinous ligament	Spinous processes of upper thoracic and mid-cervical processes to skull	Together with left and right sides or with other erectors on both sides of column, extends vertebral column and head; unilaterally side bends vertebral column
Semispinalis capitis	Tendons from C7, T6, and T7	Between inferior and superior nuchal line of occipital bone	Extends head and rotates head to opposite side of contraction

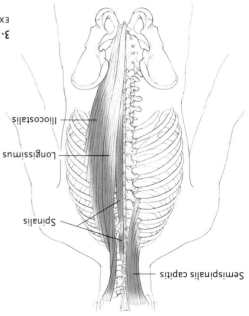

3.15   Intermediate Layer of the Extensor Muscles of the Back

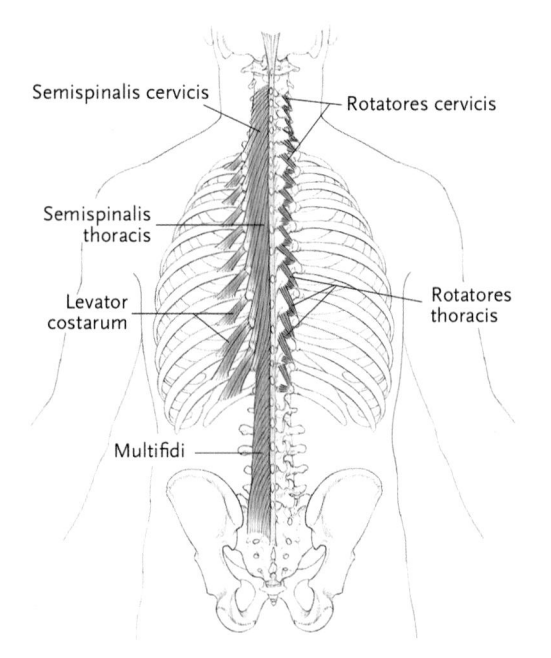

Semispinalis cervicis

Rotatores cervicis

Semispinalis thoracis

Levator costarum

Rotatores thoracis

Multifidi

3.17 DEEP LAYER OF THE EXTENSOR MUSCLES OF THE BACK

3.18   DEEP LAYER OF THE EXTENSOR MUSCLES OF THE BACK

Muscle	Origin	Insertion	Action
Semispinalis cervicis	Transverse processes of adjacent vertebrae	Spinous and transverse processes of superior vertebrae	Stabilizes vertebrae during vertebral column movement; assists in rotation and extension
Semispinalis thoracis	Transverse processes of adjacent vertebrae	Spinous and transverse processes of superior vertebrae	Stabilizes vertebrae during vertebral column movement; assists in rotation and extension
Multifidi	Transverse processes of adjacent vertebrae	Spinous and transverse processes of superior vertebrae	Stabilizes vertebrae during vertebral column movement; assists in rotation and extension
Rotatores cervicis	Transverse processes of adjacent vertebrae	Spinous and transverse processes of superior vertebrae	Stabilizes vertebrae during vertebral column movement; assists in rotation and extension
Rotatores thoracis	Transverse processes of adjacent vertebrae	Spinous and transverse processes of superior vertebrae	Stabilizes vertebrae during vertebral column movement; assists in rotation and extension
Levator costarum	Transverse processes of adjacent vertebrae	Spinous and transverse processes of superior vertebrae	Stabilizes vertebrae during vertebral column movement; assists in rotation and extension

this once, and then have her reverse this exercise, so she is lifting from the lumbar spinous processes, one by one to C1. No doubt this is difficult to feel, but it will reveal where her spine is hypomobile, that is, where she does not move well. She can continue to do this daily as both an awareness and a mobilization technique.

The spinal column is designed for movement, but it is also designed for stability. This stability is created in part by structures in the column that resemble the legs of a tripod stool. These three structures are the intervertebral disc as one leg of the stool and each of the facet joints as the other two legs. When you stand with all the normal curves undisturbed, that is, in the anatomical position, the curves are in a neutral position, and all three legs of the stool are in contact. That is the position in which the spinal column is the most stable.

To demonstrate this, have your student stand in Tadasana on a nonskid mat. Once he is aligned and after asking permission to touch him, stand behind him and firmly press down on the tops of his shoulders. If he is aligned with a perfect tripod alignment, he will withstand your pressure with no problem. However, if there is a deviation, for example, his lumbar curve is in slight flexion or slight extension, he will buckle slightly under the pressure. This is one of the easiest ways to check for the neutral alignment of the column.

When students move into asana, they distort the curves and eliminate the tripod shape. Of course, it would be impossible to move at all unless one was able to partially or completely reverse the spinal curves, rotate, and bend in all directions. But when in vertical poses like Tadasana, and when sitting, creating the neutral curves will create the most stability.

Another important aspect of the kinesiology of the vertebral column is the ROM of each segment. The ROM of each vertebral segment is determined by the intervertebral discs. If the discs are plump and full, the movement at that segment will be normal. If not, movement can be limited. The direction of movement at any vertebral segment is determined, however, by the angle of the facet joints. For example, the angle of the cervical facets is about 45 degrees. This allows for flexion and extension, side bending, and rotation. More details about the movements allowed are discussed in chapters 4, 5, 6, and 7, which deal in depth with each region of the spinal column.

The effect on the movement of the column as a whole varies with flexion and extension. In flexion, there is stress on the supraspinal ligaments, the interspinous ligaments, the ligamentum flavum, the capsule of the facet joint, the PLL, and finally on the posterior disc. In extension of the column, the stress occurs first on the ALL, then on the disc, on the joint, and finally on the spinous processes, if there is any impingement of the superior one on an inferior one.

EXPERIENTIAL ANATOMY

For Practicing

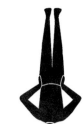

3.19
TADASANA,
WITH THE
HANDS ON
THE PELVIS

Applied Practice: Finding the Neutral Position of Your Pelvis

Prop: 1 nonskid mat

Take Care: Press lightly but firmly.

THE PELVIS is the pot out of which the spinal column grows. If the pelvis is tilted, the column is affected. Whatever sitting position you find yourself in right now, just move your pelvis in any direction only an inch and you will notice a direct effect on the column. Try it a couple of times.

To find the neutral position of your pelvis, stand on your nonskid mat in Tadasana. Put your hands around the top of the pelvis, across the tops of the ilia, so your thumb is in the back and your fingers come around to the front (Figure 3.19).

Imagine that the top ridge of your ilia (which is the spine of the ilia) is parallel to the floor. This will take a little practice because this is a curved surface, so take your time. Let your fingers feel the anterior superior iliac spine (ASIS) of the pelvis and your thumbs feel the posterior superior iliac spine (PSIS). When you think you have found the neutral position, your fingers and thumb will be about the same height from the floor. To test if this is truly the right position, press straight down hard. If your pelvis is in a neutral position, no movement will occur. If the position you selected is not the neutral one, then you will feel a movement under your hands. Please remember that this is an art as well as a concrete adjustment, so if you are unable to understand it the first time, don't be discouraged. Try it several times, until you find the position in which your pelvis is neutral.

Another way to verify that your pelvis is in a neutral position is to feel for any tension in the abdomen wall between the ASIS and the symphysis pubis. If you are in neutral, this area will feel soft; if not, it will feel taut.

For Teaching

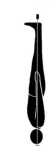

3.20
TADASANA,
WITH
PLUMB LINE

Applied Teaching: Practicing with Normal Curves in Tadasana

Prop: 1 nonskid mat

Take Care: Make sure your suggested adjustments do not create lower back discomfort for the student.

TEACHING STUDENTS to be aware of their normal spinal curves can help them, not only in asana but also in their daily life, as they sit at a desk, lift heavy packages, and stand in line.

The first concept to understand is a plumb line, which is a vertical line that you can visualize on your student's lateral side (Figure 3.20). It passes through the external auditory meatus of the ear, the center of the shoulder joint, the hip joint, the center of the knee joint, and finally the lateral malleolus of the ankle.

To help the student find this vertical awareness, have her stand in Tadasana on a nonskid mat and against a corner. When she does so, she should touch the corner at the occiput, mid-thoracic spine, distal sacrum, and superior coccyx. This aid is a little inexact but is nonetheless a good beginning to awareness.

As you help your student align herself in Tadasana, look for these additional common misalignments in the pose:

▶ Feet: Most people stand with a least one of their feet turned out. Notice the student's feet and ask her to stand in Tadasana with the outside borders of her feet parallel to the edges of her mat. Try pressing down on her shoulders with her feet in her normal position, and then follow it with pressing down with her feet parallel. Both of you will feel the difference in stability when the outside edges of her feet are parallel to the mat. This is because, in the aligned position of the feet, the tripod of the facet joints of the vertebral column is created, as well as the maximum congruence of the concave–convex surfaces of other weight-bearing joints, like the hip joints and knee joints.

▶ Knees: One of the things students do in Tadasana is to push back on their knees to the point of hyperextension of the joints. Check that your student has not done this and that the imaginary plumb line runs directly through her knee joint.

▶ Pelvis: This is critical to position correctly. After she has given you permission to touch, stand behind your student and place your hands on the top of the crest of her illia. If your hand is straight and flat, the highest portion of the crest of her illia will be parallel to the floor. With your middle finger, now feel her ASISs. Imagine these points as just touching a virtual flat plane or wall parallel to the student. If her pelvis is aligned, both of these points will be parallel with the plumb line.

▶ Scapulae: Make sure her scapulae are not winging out and are as vertical as possible. Most people carry their scapulae in a diagonal rather than a vertical line in relation to the vertebral column.

▶ Head: Stand at her side and make sure that the plumb line runs through the outer auditory meatus of her ear and that her eyes are slightly lower than the top of her ears.

You can ask your student to try Tadasana at a protruding corner of a wall, with the following parts of the body touching it: coccyx, mid-thoracic spine, and posterior midline skull. See if this aids his understanding of Tadasana and his neutral spinal curves.

LINK

Tadasana is not only important for maintaining the health of the spine but also helps to keep the abdominal organs in placc. When you stand with the normal curves intact, the organs rest on each other to form a visceral column. When the spinal curves are disturbed, the force of gravity is no longer transmitted through the organs in the most efficient way, which puts stress on them, particularly the bladder. For more information, consult *Urogenital Manipulation* by Jean-Pierre Barral (Seattle, WA: Eastland Press, 1993).

The Cervical Spine 4

ONE INTERESTING WAY to look at the posture of the cervical spine is to think of it as receiving the results of the posture of the spinal segments below it. If you slump, the neck will be affected; if you stand with your normal spinal curves in alignment, the neck will also be affected. However you choose to hold your lumbar and thoracic spines will create health or havoc for the cervical spine above them.

Head and neck posture can also signal your mood to the world. For example, you may communicate that you are feeling poised, assertive, meditative, or dejected, all by what you do with your head and neck. Poor neck posture can contribute to headaches, as well as to neck and eyestrain. Salamba Sirsasana and Salamba Sarvangasana, two of the core postures of yoga practice, depend on an awareness of and alignment in the cervical spine. Many of the problems associated with the cervical spine in asana can be avoided or solved by remembering to create and maintain a normal

cervical lordosis as much as possible in each pose (Figures 4.1 and 4.2). This is the position of least strain for the neck.

BONES

The top two cervical vertebrae are especially unique, both in structure and function. The cervical spine originates at the juncture of the skull and the first cervical vertebrae, called the skull-C1 joint. The first cervical vertebra is also called the atlas, after Atlas in Greek mythology, who holds the world on his shoulders. Like him, we hold the globe of the skull on the atlas, C1. Another name for this joint is the atlanto-occipital joint (Figure 4.3).

The first cervical joint is notable because it is the only movable vertebra that has no body. Instead it is a bony ring with flattened facet surfaces that articulate with the corresponding surfaces on the distal skull to create the joint. The union of these two

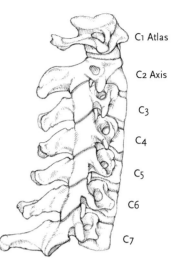

C1 Atlas

C2 Axis

C3

C4

C5

C6

C7

4.1 (RIGHT) SAGITTAL VIEW OF THE CERVICAL SPINE

4.2 (OPPOSITE LEFT) POSTERIOR VIEW OF CERVICAL SPINE, WITH EIGHT CERVICAL NERVES EXITING AND VIEW OF THE VERTEBRAL ARTERY

4.3 (OPPOSITE RIGHT) ATLAS VERTEBRAE AND AXIS VERTEBRAE, WITH SKULL AND C1 LIGAMENTS

bones is shaped somewhat like a cup and saucer, the skull being the cup and C1 being the saucer. There is no intervertebral disc between the skull and C1. Also notable is that the first cervical vertebra has no spinous process.

The second cervical vertebra is distinctive as well. During embryological development, the body of C1 migrates distally and joins the anterior body of C2 (also called the axis), creating a prominence called either the odontoid process or the dens. It is approximately ⅜ inch in height and protrudes upward into the C1 vertebrae. Like the skull and C1, there is no intervertebral disc between C1 and C2. The rest of the cervical vertebrae are more similar in construction. A unique aspect of the structure of the cervical spine is the bifid spinous process of C2 through C6. Another unusual aspect of the structure of the cervical spine is the existence of the transverse foramen. This is the opening in the transverse processes that allows for the passage of the vertebral artery, one of the two blood supplies to the brain.

It is important to understand the significance of this relationship in asana practice. The movement of the cervical spine can directly affect the blood supply to the brain. This artery can be occluded by a combination of rotation and extension. In other words, if you rotate to the right and backbend to the right you can occlude the right vertebral artery. For young people with healthy arteries, this movement is no problem. But in students over the age of sixty, it is important to pay attention to this movement. Especially pay attention to this alignment in seated twists.

Often a student will rotate the cervical spine in a seated twist, and you will notice that she tilts her head backward; be sure to suggest that she rotate her cervical spine while keeping her chin parallel to the floor instead. This will minimize any compression on the vertebral artery. Symptoms of vertebral artery compression can be dizziness and/ or a rapid back-and-forth eye movement called nystagmus.

The other source of blood and oxygen to the brain is the carotid arteries at the lateral sides of the neck. Take a moment now to find them. Turn your neck to the right about halfway. Palpate the contracted left sternocleidomastoid muscle near the jaw line. Now move your fingers slightly anteriorly, and feel the pulse of the carotid artery beneath them.

There is another bone in the cervical region: the U-shaped hyoid. It is located at the base of the tongue, at the level of the third cervical vertebra,

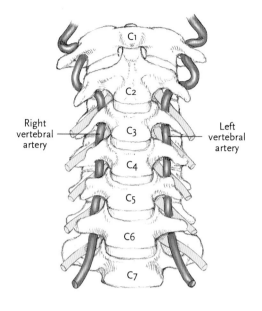

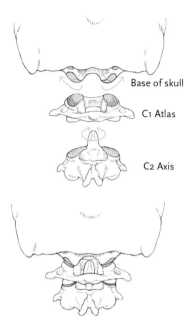

below the mandible and above the larynx. It is the origin for the tongue muscles. The hyoid is unique in that it does not articulate with any other bone; rather it is held in place by the stylo-hyoid ligaments, suspended from the styloid processes of the temporal bones. It assists in swallowing and speech.

JOINTS

Only two movements are allowed at the skull–C1 joint: flexion and extension. These movements are determined by the angle of the facet joints, as they are at all vertebral segments. This relationship is like a cup and saucer. Thus the skull–C1 joint only allows for the skull to rock backward (extension) and forward (flexion) on C1. There is no rotation allowed at this segment.

The atlanto-axial joint, or C1–C2, on the other hand, allows for flexion, extension, and rotation because the facets face in an angle of about 45 degrees. This is also true for the rest of the cervical spine as well; we discuss it in detail later in this chapter.

CONNECTIVE TISSUE

In addition to the strong ligaments that hold the skull to C1, the strongest and largest ligament in the cervical region is the ligament nuchae (see Figure 3.9 in chapter 3). You can usually palpate this ligament easily along the central portion of the cervical spine in strong cervical flexion. With your neck in flexion, place your fingers against the spinous processes in the mid-cervical region. The ligament is usually prominent in this area.

You can feel this ligament while your student is in Salamba Sarvangasana. To do this, have your student practice with at least five blankets under his shoulders and with his feet on the wall. Once he is has rolled up into the pose, he can keep his feet on the wall for safety and support. After asking permission to touch him, feel the back of his neck, focusing on the mid-cervical region to feel the ligament. It should be slightly taut, as it is under a great deal of stretch.

In the cervical region, the posterior longitudinal ligament can fold into the spinal canal on extension of the cervical spine if the intervertebral discs have

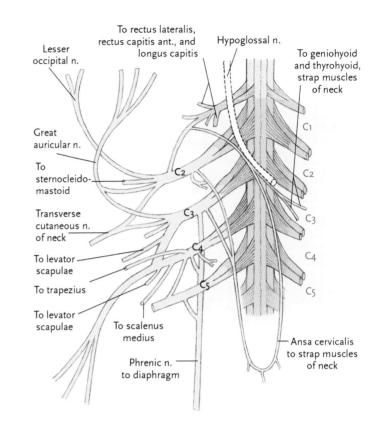

Lesser
occipital n.

To rectus lateralis,
rectus capitis ant., and
longus capitis

Hypoglossal n.

To geniohyoid
and thyrohyoid,
strap muscles
of neck

C1

C2

Great
auricular n.

To
sternocleido-
mastoid

C2

C3

Transverse
cutaneous n.
of neck

C3

C4

To levator
scapulae

C4

To trapezius

C5

C5

To levator
scapulae

To scalenus
medius

Ansa cervicalis
to strap muscles
of neck

Phrenic n.
to diaphragm

4.4 SCHEMATIC OF THE CERVICAL PLEXUS

degenerated. (See Figure 3.6 for the location of healthy structures.) This can press on nerves, causing pain and dysfunction, so this action should be approached carefully by those with cervical disc degeneration.

NERVES

As discussed in chapter 3, although there are only seven cervical vertebrae, there are eight cervical nerves, which are numbered in the same way as the vertebrae. C1 nerve exits the spinal column between the skull and C1 vertebra and is also called the suboccipital nerve. The second cervical nerve exits between C1 and C2 vertebrae, the third nerve between C2 and C3, and so forth (Figure 4.4).

This group of nerves is called the cervical plexus. It innervates spinal, neck, and upper trunk muscles, as well as the muscles of the face, throat, jaw, and diaphragm. In addition, divisions of the fifth to eighth cervical, together with the first thoracic

nerve, form the brachial plexus, which controls the muscles of the upper extremity. This latter plexus is discussed in more detail in chapter 13.

MUSCLES

The muscles of the cervical spine can be divided into several regions and layers. These are the superficial, lateral cervical, suprahyoid, infrahyoid, anterior, and lateral vertebral.

The superficial muscle is the platysma muscle, a broad and flat muscle arising from the fascia of the pectoralis major and deltoid and inserting into the mandible and the muscles around the mouth (Figure 4.5). Contraction of the platysma causes the lower lip and corner of the mouth to move laterally and inferiorly.

The lateral cervical muscles are the trapezius (see chapter 13) and the sternocleidomastoid muscle (SCM) (Figure 4.6). The sternal head arises from the manubrium of the sternum; the clavicular head

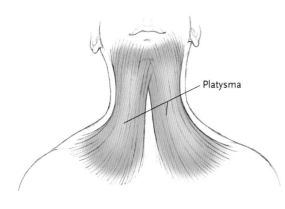

4.5 SUPERFICIAL MUSCLES OF THE CERVICAL SPINE

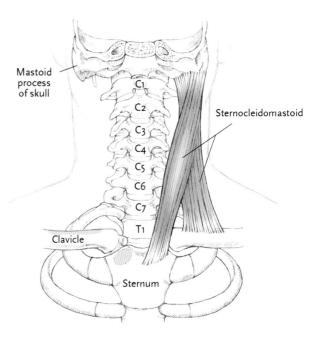

4.6 LATERAL MUSCLES OF THE CERVICAL SPINE

arises from the medial clavicle. Insertion is at the mastoid process. When contracted bilaterally, the SCM flexes the cervical spine. When contracted unilaterally, the SCM performs two actions: side bending to the same side and rotation to the opposite side.

This muscle can be clearly seen in Utthita Trikonasana. Notice your student's neck when she is practicing to the right. Her right SCM will be seen to be quite prominent, as it is contracting strongly against gravity to turn her head to the left.

The anterior vertebral muscles are the next group and are presented in the accompanying illustration and chart (Figures 4.7 and 4.8). The lateral vertebral muscles are involved with breathing and are well known to yoga students (Figures 4.9 and 4.10). When all the scalene are fixed at their origins, as a group they lift the first two ribs and thus can aid in inspiration. When the insertion is fixed, the contraction of the scalenes unilaterally side bends the cervical spine.

The anterior neck is divided at the midline into anterior and posterior triangles. The hyoid bone

divides the anterior triangle in half. The muscles of the hyoid area are the suprahyoid, stylo-hyoid, genio-hyoid, hyo-glossus, and the digastric. These muscles above the hyoid bone are involved in swallowing. The infrahyoid mucles are the infrahyoid, omo-hyoid, thyro-hyoid and sterno-thyroid. These muscles are involved in stabilizing the hyoid bone during swallowing and in making low- or high-pitched sounds.

The posterior triangle is between the trapezius and the SCM. It contains the semispinalis capitis, the levator scapulae, splenius capitis and the three scalenes.

KINESIOLOGY

A normal cervical curve is the position of least strain for all the cervical spinal structures. A healthy positioning of the cervical spine can be observed from the side in Tadasana. If your student is standing with all his spinal curves in neutral, his neck should receive the benefit of this alignment. Check this by observing the top of his ear. This should be

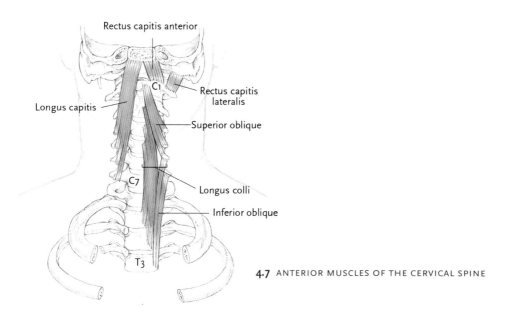

Rectus capitis anterior

C1

Longus capitis

Rectus capitis lateralis

Superior oblique

C7

Longus colli

Inferior oblique

T3

4.7 ANTERIOR MUSCLES OF THE CERVICAL SPINE

4.8 ANTERIOR MUSCLES OF THE CERVICAL SPINE

NAME	ORIGIN	INSERTION	ACTION
Longus colli	Three heads: Longitudinal: bodies of C2–C4; Superior oblique: C1; Inferior oblique: bodies of T1–T3	Longitudinal: C7–T3; Superior oblique: transverse processes of C3–C6; Inferior oblique: transverse processes of C5–C7	Unilaterally assists in side bending and rotation of head; flexes neck bilaterally
Longus capitis	Transverse processes C3–C6	Occiput anterior to rectus	Flexes head; extends upper cervical spine
Rectus capitis anterior	Mass of atlas	Occiput	Flexes head; assists in side bending and rotation
Rectus capitis lateralis	Transverse process of atlas	Jugular process of occipital bone	Side bends head

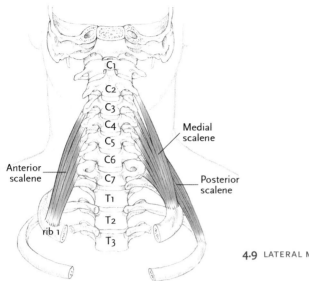

C1
C2
C3
C4
C5
C6
C7
T1
T2
T3

Medial scalene

Anterior scalene

Posterior scalene

rib 1

4.9 LATERAL MUSCLES OF THE CERVICAL SPINE

4.10 LATERAL MUSCLES OF THE CERVICAL SPINE

MUSCLE	ORIGIN	INSERTION	ACTION
Anterior scalene	Transverse processes of C3–C6	Anterior first rib	When spine is fixed, bilaterally, raises first two ribs during forced inspiration; assists neck flexion and contralateral rotation when ribs are fixed
Medial scalene	Transverse processes of C2–C7	Cranial surface of first rib	When spine is fixed, bilaterally, raises first two ribs during forced inspiration; assists neck flexion and contralateral rotation when ribs are fixed
Posterior scalene	Transverse processes of C4–C6	Second rib	When spine is fixed, bilaterally, raises first two ribs during forced inspiration; assists neck flexion and contralateral rotation when ribs are fixed; especially aids in side bending

slightly higher than the eye. In your mind, draw a line from the top of his ear to the top of the eye socket, and make sure he is carrying his head with his eye slightly dropped. Most people do not do this; they stand with the chin higher.

The opposite of this healthy head posture, actually carrying the head forward of the body in a forward head posture, can affect every bodily system, not just the neck itself (Figure 4.11). For example, when you hold your head in the forward head posture, you also slump and round your thoracic spine. This can interfere with breathing, digestion, and elimination. I have even heard the case of a woman who had tachycardia (rapid heart rate) because her head position was interfering with the vagal nerve and its control of the heart rate. Changing her head position resolved the problem. Teaching your students to carry the head over the body will no doubt contribute to their overall health.

As stated previously, the only movements allowed between the skull and C_1 joint are flexion and extension. Thus this joint could be called the "yes joint" because its function is necessary in order for you to nod your head. But this nodding is very small.

You can experience this slight nodding when you perform the following. Sit or stand with your vertebral column in its normal curves. Pay special attention to the position of your head and neck. When you are satisfied that your cervical spine is in neutral, drop and then lift the chin about an inch or less. Repeat this movement back and forth, back and forth, flexion and extension. Try closing your eyes to concentrate more. Be sure that these movements are small. You will probably be able to feel the isolated movement at the skull and C_1.

The next joint, C_1–C_2, allows flexion, extension, and rotation, in part because of the additional structure of the dens. Thus C_1–C_2 is called the "no joint" because it allows us to shake the head from side to side. In fact, the first 50 percent of rotation

in the cervical spine comes from the C_1–C_2 joint. The additional cervical rotation is created by the remaining cervical joints, also called the lower cervicals.

This is important to understand. To feel this movement more clearly, lightly place the four fingers (not the thumb) of your right hand along the spinous processes of your cervical spine. Your little fingertip will be near your hairline and your index fingertip close to your shoulders.

Now slowly turn your head to the right. You will notice that about halfway into the rotation, the lower cervicals suddenly kick in and rotate to the left. This means the bodies of the cervical vertebrae are rotating to the right, what we call right rotation. Try it again with your left fingertips for left rotation.

This understanding will help you know what part of the cervical spine is dysfunctional if a student comes to class with the complaint that she can turn her head to one side about halfway and then it hurts or gets stuck. It will tell you that she has a misalignment in her lower cervicals. If, on the other hand, she cannot rotate her head to one side at all without pain or difficulty, then you know that the problem is with the C_1–C_2 joint.

Another important kinesiological point to understand about the cervical spine is the apex of extension and flexion in the lower cervical spine. Once again place your fingertips lightly on the spinous processes of your cervical spine; now extend your neck. Note where your feel the apex, or deepest point of the curve of the extension movement. Keep your fingertips there and perform flexion of the cervical spine. You will note that the apex of flexion moves down a vertebral level.

This is because the apex of extension is at C_4, while the apex of flexion is one segment lower at C_5. The apex is the point where the curve of the movement is the greatest. Thus the point of wear and tear for the cervical spine is at C_4 for extension and C_5 for flexion. If people have pain from cer-

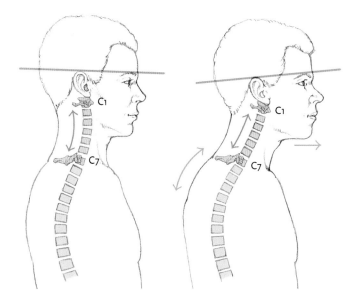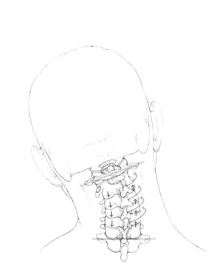

4.11 (LEFT) NORMAL CERVICAL CURVE;
(RIGHT) FORWARD HEAD, SAGITTAL VIEW

4.12 SIDE BENDING AND ROTATION, POSTERIOR VIEW

vical problems like herniated discs, they usually have it at the level of C4–C5.

How the Neck Moves. One way to understand the movement of the spinal column is to visualize it as two long series of facet joints—one right, one left. In the cervical spine, these facet joints lie in the frontal plane, at an approximate angle of 45 degrees.

To get a sense of this, hold your hands in front of your face, palms facing you. Now tilt your fingers away from you so that your hands are in a 45-degree angle to the floor. With your hands in this position, it is easy to see how the facet joints could move forward and up, as well as down and back. The forward and up movement creates flexion of the cervical spine, and the down and back sliding of the facet joints creates extension. If on one side of the spine, for example, the facets on the right side of the spine move forward and up while those on the left move down and back, the result is a left rotation. Side bending is a special type of rotation.

The general rule of side bending and rotation for the cervical spine is this: in the cervical region,

side bending and rotation occur to the same side, regardless of the position of the cervical spine at the beginning of the movement. For example, when you side bend to the left, the bodies of the vertebrae also rotate to the left. In other words, as the bodies rotate right, the spinous processes are pointing left (Figure 4.12).

You can feel this for yourself. Once again place your fingers lightly on your cervical spinous processes. Now side bend to the left; you will notice that your spinous processed rotate to the right. This means that the bodies have rotated left. While this may seem a little confusing at first, practice it for a few days and the principle will become clearer.

There is one exception to the law of side bending and rotation in the cervical spine. Notice this: when you side bend the neck to the right, we know your cervical bodies rotate right as well. But if this is true, then when you side bend right, why does your face still face forward? In other words, if the law is true, you would expect your face to turn down to the right. This does not happen and here's why.

The law is true but there is an exception. It is this: the law is that side bending and rotation are to the same side in the cervical spine except for C1-C2, which rotates the opposite way. This accomplishes keeping the face forward during side bending.

Therefore if you have a problem with side bending right, the cause could be one of the following: a restriction of side bending right, a restriction of rotation right, or a restriction of rotation left of the atlas on the axis. It is worth the time to study these principles because understanding side bending and rotation will help you understand scoliosis, the lateral curvature of the vertebral column, which is discussed in detail in chapter 6.

The law of side bending and rotation is an attempt to describe the natural movements of the cervical spine. We can all override this law by purposely choosing another action. But it is likely that when we do, there may be discomfort.

Finally, a word about neck rolls. Many yoga teachers teach their students to roll their head and neck around in a circle, first one way and then the other, to stretch the neck. But this is a nonanatomical movement and is not recommended. Remember that the cervical facets are flattened surfaces that move either forward and up or down and back. The cervical joints are not ball-and-socket joints, like the hip joints or, to a lesser extent, like the shoulder joints. When you attempt to use the cervical spine as if it were a ball-and-socket joint, in a portion of the movement the joint is gapped to the side in a nonanatomical movement.

Instead of asking your students to do neck rolls, have them move the neck in one direction at a time. For example, ask them to rotate right and hold and breathe, then rotate a little more and breathe, and so on. It is fine to have them side bend with the same instructions. They can also turn the chin down toward one shoulder and then the other, as well as the more obvious movements of flexion and extension. But neck rolls are not indicated because of the structural shape of the cervical facets.

EXPERIENTIAL ANATOMY

For Practicing

Applied Practice: Head Position in Utthita Trikonasana
Prop: 1 nonskid mat
Take Care: Do not try this if you have pre-existing cervical pain.
ALL LEVELS of students have experienced discomfort in the neck in Utthita Trikonasana at one time or another. The probable reason is that rotating the head upward in this pose does not follow the law of side bending and rotation. Thus it puts strain on the neck, as the added weight of gravity is added to the 20-pound weight of the head. When you are practicing this pose to the right, you are usually instructed to rotate your head to the left, or upward, and many students then notice discomfort, if not pain, at the base of the skull as they hold the rotation.

In the pose, you are initially side bending right, as shown previously in Figure 4.12. This is then slightly changed as you lift your head up a bit to keep it parallel to the floor. Now you are side bending left in the cervical spine, while practicing Utthita Trikonasana to the right (Figure 4.13). According to the law of side bending and rotation for the cervical

4.13
UTTHITA
TRIKONASANA

spine, when you rotate right, you side bend right but C1–C2 turns the opposite way. Thus when rotating the cervical spine left in a right Utthita Trikonasana, you are overriding the rotation at C1–C2, which would ordinarily be to the right. Overcoming this natural tendency against the force of gravity can cause discomfort. If you have not felt this discomfort, then hold the pose longer and you will. Another suggestion is to practice the pose with the face forward, to minimize discomfort at the upper cervical region.

For Teaching

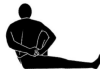

4.14
MARICHY-
ASANA III

Applied Teaching 1: The Cervical Spine in Twists
Prop: 1 nonskid mat
Take Care: To protect the lower back, make sure that the student twists his pelvis with his whole spine in this pose and does not hold it stationary.
When your student practices a seated twist like Marichyasana III, notice his cervical spine from the back (Figure 4.14). As he twists to the right, the right side of the neck will shorten and the left will lengthen, according to the law. He is rotating right and thus is side bending right. If you measure carefully, the right side of his neck will indeed be shorter.

If the C1-C2 joint is functioning properly, his head will remain level because this joint rotates in the opposite way. If not, then you will notice that he is tilting his head back and to the right. This is a sign that there is a dysfunction at C1-C2.

4.15
SALAMBA
SIRSASANA

Applied Teaching 2: The Cervical Spine in Salamba Sirsasana
Props: 1 nonskid mat • 1 blanket
Take Care: Your student should avoid this pose if she has pre-existing neck pain; numbness, tingling, or radiating pain in her arms; osteoporosis of the spine; high blood pressure; pressure in her eyes; or if she is menstruating, pregnant, or more than 25 pounds overweight.
When the student practices Salamba Sirsasana, observe her cervical spine from the side first (Figure 4.15). Notice if she is maintaining the normal cervical curve. Do this by making sure that the base of her skull is in a vertical line with her C7 vertebrae. Her chin should be level with the floor, not dropping or lifting. Notice if her neck looks too flat.

Now move to her back. There should be an even gully down the middle of her posterior neck. If the cervical curve is too flat, these gullies will not appear. If this is the case, she needs to move slowly toward her forehead so she creates the natural curve.

Applied Teaching 3: The Cervical Spine in Salamba Sarvangasana and Halasana
Props: 1 nonskid mat • 6 firm blankets, each folded into a shape of 12 x 21 x 28 inches
Take Care: Students should avoid this pose if they have pre-existing neck pain; numbness, tingling, or radiating pain in her arms; osteoporosis of the spine; high blood

pressure; pressure in the eyes; or if they are menstruating, pregnant, or more than 25 pounds overweight.

As we have seen, the key to a healthy cervical spine is maintaining the normal cervical curve. This is virtually impossible to do while practicing Salamba Sarvangasana and Halasana. But protecting the cervical spine is important. If students stretch the soft tissues of the posterior cervical spine the maximum amount and then put the weight of the body on it, it can be not only challenging to the cervical spine but also potentially damaging.

To protect the cervical spine in Salamba Sarvangasana, I recommend placing firm blankets (folded as noted) under the shoulders to lift them at least 6 to 8 inches from the floor, so the cervical spine is at an angle of about 120 degrees (Figure 4.16). This is appropriate because there is only about 60 to 70 degrees of flexion allowed in the cervical spine normally. Any more of an angle than that would not only be forcing the cervical spine beyond its natural abilities but would also tend to recruit upper thoracic joints into too much flexion. The weight bearing of this pose is to be done on the shoulders and not on the cervical or thoracic spines.

Another way to ascertain if your student's cervical spine is in too much flexion is to check the ligamentum nuchae. After asking permission, gently touch the back of your student's neck while he is in Salamba Sarvangasana. Note how tight the ligament feels. If it is extremely tight and taut under your hands, he probably needs more height under his shoulders.

Halasana causes a strong flattening of the cervical spine, even more than Salamba Sarvangasana. Therefore, if the student already has a tight ligamentum nuchae in Salamba Sarvangasana, Halasana will cause additional strain to the structures of the cervical spine. Add even more height under his shoulders to protect his neck.

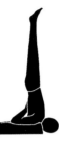

4.16
SALAMBA
SARVANG-
ASANA

Applied Teaching 4: The Cervical Spine in Back Bends
Props: 1 chair • 2 nonskid mats • 1 blanket
Take Care: Do not practice this pose if there is pre-existing neck pain; radiating pain, numbness, or tingling in your arms; or lower back pain when practicing.
One of the most well-known back bends is Bhujangasana (Figure 4.17). Part of the pose involves extension of the cervical spine. But notice how some students practice this pose: they appear to back bend the neck, but really they are in cervical flexion, while back bending only the upper cervical spine.

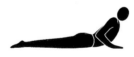

4.17
BHUJANG-
ASANA,
LATERAL VIEW

To understand how this works, try this. While sitting, slightly flex your neck so that you are looking down. Now back bend from the top of your cervical spine only, by lifting your chin a few inches. Note how your lower cervicals are in flexion, while your upper cervical spine is in extension. This is not true extension, and it is common for students to do this in Bhujangasana.

To practice Bhujangasana, have your student lie on a nonskid mat, with a blanket on top for comfort (if desired) and another mat, folded in fours, placed under the abdomen. Position the legs about 12 inches apart, and internally rotate them. Place the hands on the floor, so the fingertips are under the tops of the shoulders. As the student exhales, she lifts up into an arch, primarily using the back to lift and minimizing the help from the arms. She should continue to breathe normally in the pose. Students can also practice this pose with their arms out to the sides (so the body forms a T-shape) or with the arms stretched back alongside the body and slightly lifted.

Make sure that students practice an even extension in this pose, by keeping the top of the head facing the opposite wall instead of stretching the chin outward.

LINK

During seated pranayama, students frequently include the practice of Jalandhara Bandha, or chin lock. In this position, the cervical spine is in full flexion. Please remember that the greatest reversal of the cervical curve occurs when the chin is tucked in first before flexion occurs. Make sure that when your students practice Jalandhara Bandha, they first flex the cervical spine and then draw the chin in to create the lock. This will lessen the stress on the cervical spine.

The Thoracic Spine and Rib Cage 5

THE THORACIC SPINE is a unique part of the vertebral column. It helps to create the posterior armature of the thoracic cage, serves as an attachment point for the ribs, and provides a strong protective structure for the heart and lungs.

The normal thoracic curve is convex posteriorly, the opposite of the cervical spine, and is more stable than the neck, allowing less range of movement. This is generally true in the body. As one descends the skeleton, there is less mobility but more stability; as one ascends, there is more mobility but less stability in the weight-bearing joints.

BONES

The thorax consists of the sternum, ribs, and costal cartilage anteriorly and laterally, and the thoracic spine posteriorly (Figure 5.1).

The mostly flat sternum, or breastbone, is made up of three bones. The most superior one is the

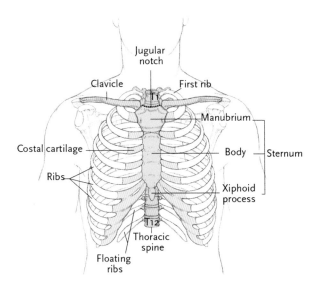

5.1 THORACIC SPINE, ANTERIOR VIEW

manubrium, which has a notch at the superior border called the jugular notch. This is the place where the chin rests during Jalandhara Bandha, or chin lock, during pranayama practice. At the sides and top of the manubrium are surfaces for the articula-

65

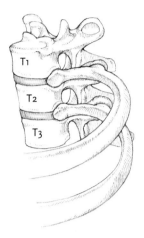

5.2 THORACIC SPINE, WITH DEMIFACETS AND RIBS;
POSTERIOR VIEW

tion of the sternum with the clavicle and with the first rib.

Take a moment to palpate this area on yourself. Place your fingertips at the base of your throat and at the top of your sternum. Feel gently the V-shaped jugular notch. Now move your fingers to one side, and find the location where the manubrium and clavicle join. This is the sternoclavicular joint.

The next part of the sternum is the body. This is the largest and longest portion of the sternum. At the point where the manubrium and body join is the sternal angle. The second rib joins the sternum at the sternal angle. In adults, the sternum is a key site of blood cell production.

The sternum typically ends in the xiphoid process, although not all people have one. During youth it is cartilaginous but is completely ossified by the age of twenty-five. The xiphoid process serves as an attachment for the rectus abominus muscle. (See chapter 11 for more details on this muscle.) Finally, the sternum articulates on either side, not only with the clavicle but also with the cartilage of the first seven ribs.

The ribs make up another major structure of the thorax. There are twenty-four ribs, which attach posteriorly to the thoracic vertebrae, T1-T12 (Figure 5.2). Anteriorly ribs 3-7 articulate directly with the body of the sternum by costal cartilage. These are sometimes called true ribs. These ribs attach to vertebrae T1-T 7. Remember that the first rib passes under the clavicle, not above.

The rest of the five pairs are called false ribs because they are not directly connected to the sternum. Instead, cartilage attaches the first three of these pairs to cartilage, which does attach to the sternum. The final two pairs are termed floating ribs because they are only attached to the thoracic spine and not to anything on the other end. Thus ribs T8-T12 attach to the corresponding vertebrae above and below.

Each individual rib is made up of several parts, including a head. The head of the rib is enlarged and has two articular surfaces, which join with the bodies of the two adjacent vertebrae. In other words, as the rib curves anteriorly, it touches two vertebrae. This union between vertebrae and rib is called a demifacet, which is a synovial joint.

The spinous processes of the thoracic spine vary by groups of four (Figure 5.3). The first four thoracic spinous processes point posteriorly in a fairly horizontal angle. The next set of four, numbers five through eight, point almost straight down. This directional shape of the spinous processes creates greater stability at the mid-thoracic region by limiting the movement of extension. This limitation increases protection for the heart posteriorly. The final four thoracic spinous processes point slightly more distally than the first four but more horizontally that the middle ones.

Yoga students sometimes suffer from back bender's rib. This is a rotational fault of a thoracic vertebra caused during back bending. Because the spinous processes in the mid-region are less mobile than the other thoracic vertebrae, during extension (back bending) they may not glide as easily as other thoracic vertebrae. Sometimes, when the student continues with strong extension movements, instead of the mid-thoracic vertebra extending on the one below it, it slightly rotates instead. This causes the attached ribs to rotate and creates discomfort. Often this discomfort is experienced when the student takes a deep breath. If this happens, I recommend a consultation with a health care professional.

JOINTS

The superior thoracic vertebral facets of the vertebrae face posteriorly, in an almost vertical plane; the inferior facets thus face anteriorly. The almost vertical angle of these facets allows for a great deal of movement, although less than in the cervical spine. Side bending is practically free, up to 45 degrees, and is only limited by the sternum and ribs. This free side bending is what creates the main movement of Utthita Trikonasana.

The angle of the thoracic facets also allows for 45-degree rotation. Remember that rotation can be thought of as the facets on one side of the spine moving forward and up and the facets on the other side moving down and back. Flexion is limited by the posterior ligaments and muscles; as stated before, extension is limited by the spinous processes. The site of greatest mobility is the T8-T9 joint. The superior facet surfaces of the twelfth thoracic vertebra are similar in orientation to those of all thoracic vertebrae. In other words, the superior facets of T12 face posteriorly. Thus the top portion of the T12 vertebra is thoracic in orientation. The inferior facets of T12, however, are like the rest of the lumbar facets, in that they face laterally.

Because T11 and T12 are the most like the lumbar facets, they allow the greatest amount of flexion and extension in the thoracic spine.

You will recall that the facet surfaces on the bodies of the thoracic vertebrae connect one to another. In addition there is a demifacet on the vertebral bodies, which is the site of the articulation of the ribs with the vertebrae. One of these is near the root of the pedicle on the superior portion of the vertebrae, and the other near the vertebral notch at the

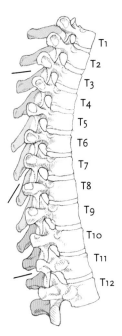

5.3 THORACIC SPINE, WITH THE THREE SECTIONS OF SPINOUS PROCESSES; SAGITTAL VIEW

inferior portion of the body. These joints between the thoracic vertebral bodies and the rib are synovial joints.

Finally, it should be remembered that the cervical-thoracic intersection is a unique joint. It is called a transitional segment because the superior facets of the first thoracic vertebrae are more like the cervical facets, and the inferior vertebral facets are more like the other thoracic facets. This is the site where the cervical lordosis begins to change into the thoracic kyphosis. Thus it is the site of possible strain. It is a good idea to make sure that this area is protected by attention to the upright posture. When your student maintains Tadasana in this area, she reduces strain on all the soft tissue in the area, like ligaments, tendons, discs, and other connective tissue, such as the capsule.

CONNECTIVE TISSUE

The ligaments of the thoracic spine are discussed in detail in chapter 3. In addition, however, the thorax is unique because of the existence of costal cartilage, which joins the ribs to the sternum.

The costal cartilages are made up of hyaline cartilage, which in effect makes the ribs longer. The first seven ribs are connected by costal cartilage directly to the sternum. The next three ribs are joined by cartilage to the lower border of the rib just above it. The last two pair of ribs are tipped with cartilage but float independently.

Another important structure in this area is the thoraco-lumbar fascia. This is a vast fascial complex that is most easily understood as connecting the last posterior ribs with the posterior iliac crest, the transverse abdominus muscle, and the transverse processes of the lumbar vertebrae, although it is connected more widely across the back. It is superficial to the quadratus lumborum muscle and can be felt by many students during forward bend practice along their back waist area. The sensation of stretching this fascial sheath is described by students as broad, flat, and superficial, as opposed to the sensation of stretching muscles, which is said to be narrow, deep, and specific.

NERVES

There are twelve thoracic nerves that exit the spinal column in this region. The first eleven pair are called intercostals and are located, as their name suggests, between the ribs. The last pair is called the subcostal and lies below the last rib.

All give off cutaneous and muscular branches. They run from the back to the front, just below each respective rib. The lower six pass into the abdominal wall, supplying, in part, the skin. The branches to the muscles control the intercostals, the abdominal muscles, and various muscles of the upper back.

MUSCLES

The extensor muscles of the thorax, or posterior paravertebral muscles, are presented in chapter 3. The flexors and rotators of the thorax are the abdominal muscles that are presented in chapter 11. The unique muscles of the thorax are the intercostal muscles.

The external intercostals arise from the lower border of the rib and attach on the upper border of the rib below; they are at right angles to the internal intercostals. The internal intercostals arise from the ridge on the inner surface of a rib and the costal cartilage and insert down and back into the superior border of the rib below, perpendicular to that rib.

The action of these muscles is to draw the ribs together, as well as to aid in inhalation and exhalation. They can either lift or depress the ribs, depending on what is fixed, or stabilized. If the last rib is held firm by the quadratus lumborum muscle, then the contraction of the intercostals will depress the rib cage and can aid in a forced exhalation. They also preserve the shape of the thoracic cage.

KINESIOLOGY

One of the unfortunate actions that sometimes happens in asana practice is an over-flattening of the natural kyphosis. Students are sometimes taught to lift the sternum with the intention of opening the chest, and they do so by bringing their thoracic spine into the body, thus flattening the curve. After years of practice, the spine loses some of its natural curve.

If this happens to you, try this. Stand on your nonskid mat, placed near a doorway. Then hold onto the edge of the doorway, with your arms at chest level and your hands crossed at the wrist. Now walk backward slowly, rounding the thoracic spine upward and encouraging your scapulae to part and move toward the sides. You should drop your head between your arms. The stretch will be felt between and under the scapulae. This stretch will help loosen some of the muscles necessary to maintain a normal kyphotic curve in the thorax.

Law of Side Bending and Rotation in the Thoracic Spine. The law of side bending and rotation in the thoracic spine is that side bending and rotation occur to the opposite side, except when the movements are begun in flexion; then they occur to the same side. For example, when you rotate your thoracic spine to the right, you side bend to the left.

Try this. Sitting in a chair, with your feet on the floor and your spine long, rotate to the right. This means the bodies of the vertebrae rotate to the right. According to the law, the thoracic spine side bends to the left. After the rotation, place your left hand on the left side of your ribs and feel the left side bend.

It is also true that when you side bend the thoracic spine to the right, it rotates to the left. To feel this, sit tall and then side bend to the right, while keeping your hand placed around the middle of the sides of your rib cage. Notice how your rib cage rotates *away* from the side bend.

In Utthita Trikonasana performed to the right, the thoracic spine and cage rotate to the left, or toward the ceiling. Thus the law of side bending and rotation enhances the natural movement we want the student to feel in the pose of turning the chest upward.

There is a different effect of the law in Parivrtta Trikonasana, however. If you start from standing and rotate first before flexing and bending down in the pose, the rotation and side bending will be to the opposite side. This means that you will be less able to drop your top ribs in the completed pose.

Remember, if you rotate right as you come into the pose, you are side bent left; this means your top or right ribs in the pose are lifted and not dropped, the way the pose is taught. However, if you turn toward the front leg first, then flex, the exception to the rule holds. This means that if you bend forward or flex over your front leg first, then rotate into the twist of Parivrtta Trikonasana, not only will you follow the law but you will practice the pose by dropping the top ribs down.

EXPERIENTIAL ANATOMY

For Practicing

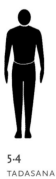

5.4
TADASANA

Applied Practice: Neutral Position of the Sternum
Props: 1 nonskid mat • 1 blanket
Take Care: Remember not to reverse your thoracic curve in an attempt to lift your sternum.
To ASCERTAIN the neutral position of the sternum, stand in Tadasana on your nonskid mat (Figure 5.4). Remember that your sternum is not a vertical bone but instead sits at an angle. The distal end of the sternum moves away from the body, while the proximal end is deeper. Try standing in Tadasana with your sternum at different angles. When the sacrum is sitting in a neutral position, your lower ribs will be in line with your anterior superior iliac spines (ASISs) and not sticking out past them, and your thoracic spine will have its neutral curve.

For Teaching

5.5
MARICHY-
ASANA III

Applied Teaching: The Thoracic Spine in Twists

Prop: 1 nonskid mat

Take Care: To protect the lower back, make sure that students twist the pelvis with the whole spine in Marichyasana III and do not hold it stationary.

REMEMBER THAT the facets in the thoracic spine allow for a great deal of rotation. However, this rotation is maximized when initiated with the spine in a neutral position. Have your student practice Marichyasana III on a nonskid mat (Figure 5.5). Notice her thoracic spine. Most students tend to flex the thoracic spine in twists. Suggest that she think of back bending her thoracic spine in the pose, which will not only bring her back to a more neutral position but also will allow her a fuller range of motion in the twist.

LINK

A useful visual aid for studying the vertebral column is a life-size model of the spine. A good source for ordering one of the many variations of vertebral models available is the Anatomical Chart Company, www.anatomical.com.

The Lumbar Spine 6

THERE ARE CERTAIN MOMENTS WHEN, WHATEVER BE THE ATTITUDE
OF THE BODY, THE SOUL IS ON ITS KNEES. —VICTOR HUGO

PROBABLY EVERY ADULT human has experienced at least one episode of lower back pain. Most of these occurrences are not serious, but this discomfort can interfere with asana practice as well as with the activities of daily living. Understanding the structure of the lumbar spine can give you the information necessary to practice and teach healthy back habits, thus preventing future pain. Understanding the lumbar spine will also help you know what to do when your back does hurt.

The lumbar spine is designed to function best as a weight-bearing structure when the lumbar curve is in its neutral position. In neutral, the lumbar spine can bear weight on the body of the vertebrae and the facet joints in a more equal and stable way. As with a three-legged stool, when all three legs are on the floor there is stability.

Remember that the lumbar spine normally has its concavity posteriorly. Many people in our culture have lost the awareness of this curve due, in part, to sitting hours each day, and in chairs that favor flexion (the flattening of the curve). Not only does maintaining the normal lumbar curve benefit the health of the lumbar spine itself, it also effects the positioning of the sacrum, which is discussed in chapter 7.

BONES

The lumbar spine consists of five massive, kidney-shaped vertebrae. The bodies of these vertebrae are wider at the transverse diameter than at the anterior-posterior one. Their main job is to bear the weight of the trunk, including the head, as well as the cervical and thoracic vertebrae (Figures 6.1 and 6.2).

The spinous processes are horizontal, large, and blunt. The transverse processes point laterally, the L3 transverse process being the widest.

The superior facet surfaces in the lumbar spine face medially, and the inferior surfaces

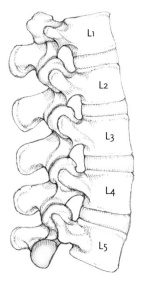

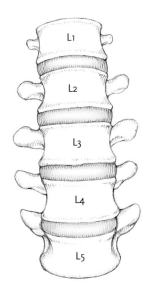

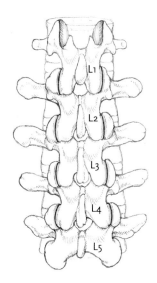

6.1 LUMBAR SPINE, SAGITTAL VIEW   **6.2** LUMBAR SPINE, ANTERIOR VIEW   **6.3** LUMBAR SPINE, POSTERIOR VIEW

face laterally. Thus these facet surfaces are almost vertical in orientation and therefore lie in the sagittal plane. To facilitate your understanding of lumbar movement, study the angle of the lumbar facets in Figure 3.5 (see chapter 3) and Figure 6.3.

Joints

The facet joints in the lumbar spine are similar in structure to each other, with the exception of the superior facet surfaces at the T12-L1 joint and the inferior facet surfaces at the L5-S1 joint.

A similar variation is true of the L5 vertebra (Figure 6.4). The superior facets of L5 are like the rest of the lumbar facets, in that they face medially. But the inferior facets of L5 face anteriorly so that they can catch on the posteriorly facing superior facet of S1 vertebra. This contributes more stability to the L5-S1 joint.

Connective Tissue

As discussed in chapter 3, the lumbar spine has three important ligaments. The first is the anterior longitudinal ligament (ALL), running from axis to sacrum along the anterior surface of the bodies (Figure 6.5). It is one of the strongest ligaments in the body. As such, it resists the weight of the lumbar spine from moving anteriorly and therefore acts as a limitation to extension. Thus, in the lumbar region, the ALL is significant in maintaining the curves not only of the lumbar as the base of the column but also essentially of the entire vertebral column.

The next is the posterior longitudinal ligament (PLL), which runs along the posterior side of the spinal canal, connecting the bodies of the vertebrae (Figure 6.5). In flexion of the column, it helps to increase pressure on the blood supply to the vertebral bodies, thus trapping fluid in the bodies and increasing their ability to bear weight. However, in the lumbar region, the PLL narrows considerably and so does not give as much support to the intervertebral discs in the lumbar as elsewhere.

The third ligament is the supraspinous ligament, which attaches the points of the spinous processes from C7 to the sacrum. It is stretched on forward bending and twists and slack on back bending. The PLL and the supraspinous ligaments

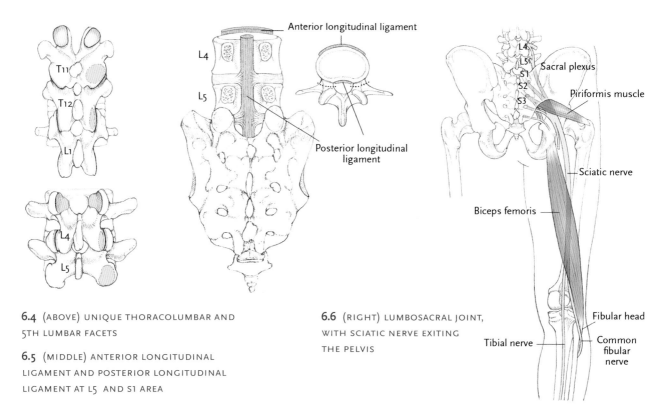

6.4 (ABOVE) UNIQUE THORACOLUMBAR AND 5TH LUMBAR FACETS

6.5 (MIDDLE) ANTERIOR LONGITUDINAL LIGAMENT AND POSTERIOR LONGITUDINAL LIGAMENT AT L5 AND S1 AREA

6.6 (RIGHT) LUMBOSACRAL JOINT, WITH SCIATIC NERVE EXITING THE PELVIS

give resistance to flexion and absorb the posterior movement of the nuclei of the discs.

NERVES

As described in chapter 3, the structure of the spinal cord in the lumbar region is unique. The spinal cord ends in the lumbar region and becomes a group of nerve fibers called the cauda equina, or horse's tail, which continues to course down the body (see Figure 3.10 in chapter 3). At the end of the cauda equina is a structure called the filum terminale, which attaches to the first segment of the coccyx.

Two major nerve plexes (groups of nerves) are involved in the lumbar region. The first is the lumbar plexus, which is formed from the L1-L4 nerve roots and from variable contribution from the T12 nerve root. This plexus sits posterior to the psoas major muscle or is intertwined with its fibers. These lumbar nerve roots control some parts of the organs of the lower abdominal wall. The L1-L4 nerves control the muscles of the anterior thigh,

parts of the medial leg, and the cutaneous innervation in this area.

The second plexus is the sacral plexus. It consists of nerves from roots L4, L5, S1, S2, and S3 (Figure 6.6). These nerves join together into one large, flat nerve root, about as big around as the index finger. This structure is called the sciatic nerve, the largest and longest nerve in the body, and it leaves the pelvis through the greater sciatic notch, which is found midway between the greater trochanter and the ischial tuberosity. After passing through the notch, it continues distally, leaving the pelvis to lie under the piriformis muscle. In some cases, the nerve is intertwined with the piriformis muscle. At the back of the thigh, it lies under the long head of the biceps femoris, one of the hamstring muscles. Finally it splits above the back of the knee. One part continues directly down the back of the calf and is called the tibial nerve. The other branch is the common peroneal nerve; it winds around the fibular head, dividing as it courses down the lateral and anterior leg.

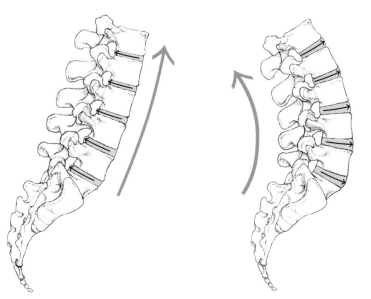

6.7 (LEFT) LUMBAR FLEXION, WITH EFFECT ON INTERVERTEBRAL DISC

6.8 (RIGHT) LUMBAR EXTENSION, WITH EFFECT ON INTERVERTEBRAL DISC

The sciatic nerve and/or its branches supply the muscles of the posterior thigh. Its branches (like the saphenous nerve) supply some or all of the cutaneous innervation of the skin below the knee as well. (Note: L4 and L5 nerves make up part of the lumbar plexus as well as part of the sacral plexus.)

MUSCLES

The flexors of the lumbar spine are the abdominal muscles as well as the short hip flexors, which are the psoas major, psoas minor, and iliacus. The abdominals are discussed in detail in chapter 11. The hip flexors are presented in chapter 8. The lumbar extensors were discussed in chapter 3. Side bending and rotation are created by the actions of the flexors and extensors; side bending and rotation are discussed in the following section.

KINESIOLOGY

The lower back is an area of discomfort for many people. To improve your yoga practice and teaching, spend some time studying how it moves based on its unique structure.

Movements Allowed in the Lumbar Spine. As discussed in chapter 3, the direction of movement in any vertebral segment is controlled by the angle of the facet joints in that region. The lumbar facets rest in the sagittal plane. Therefore the only significant movements allowed in this region are flexion and extension. In fact, flexion and extension are relatively free, limited in large part by soft tissue.

Adding up all the degrees of movement of flexion allowed in the entire vertebral column, 50 percent of that movement is created in the lumbar spine. Of that, some 75 percent is created at the L5-S1 joint. Thus 37.5 percent of all vertebral flexion occurs at one joint segment (Figure 6.7). It is no surprise then, given the vulnerable position of the fifth lumbar vertebra and the amount of flexion allowed, that this joint would be the site of frequent dysfunction. Remember that the fifth lumbar sits at an angle such that it is partially tipped forward by its connection to the angled sacrum and partially pulled in a more vertical position by its connection with L4 and the other lumbar vertebrae. Gravity is pulling L5 forward, and yet it lacks the support of a wide PLL. Add to this the extreme freedom in its range of motion in flexion, and it makes sense that the L5 disc would be subject to unusual strains.

Extension in the lumbar is basically limited by the ALL and the abdominal muscles and organs. The facets in this region actually allow for an almost complete free range of extension (Figure 6.8). However, rotation in the lumbar spine is quite limited. Although it may seem like you are rotating from your lumbar spine in a seated twist, this is not really happening because rotation is so limited in the lumbar spine.

Picture a dresser drawer: It only moves in and out; it cannot move from side to side. The lumbar spine is similar. Because of the vertical angle of the facet joints, sideways movement is minimized. There is about 12 degrees of rotation allowed at L4-L5 and the least amount of rotation in all the lumbar spine of about 6 degrees at L5-S1. The overall average of rotation in the lumbar spine is about 10 degrees.

Side bending is allowed in the lumbar spine and is about 35 degrees. It is limited by the ribs, pelvis, and soft tissue (Figure 6.9).

Law of Side Bending and Rotation in the Lumbar Spine. Here side bending and rotation occur to the opposite side, except when the movements are begun in flexion; then they occur to the same side. This means that when you twist to the right, your lumbar vertebral bodies twist right as you bend left.

Try this experiment. Sit on the edge of a chair with your vertebral column in neutral. Exhale and twist to the right. When you do so, you will notice your left side ribs bending slightly to the left. It is possible to override this movement, but if you let the twist happen naturally, you will feel the side bend. Another way to understand this law is in Utthita Trikonasana. When practicing to the right, you are side bending right. The law states that you will thus be rotating left. This is what you experience in the pose when you turn the chest upward: right side bend and left rotation. Remember that there is not much rotation allowed in the lumbar spine, but there is some.

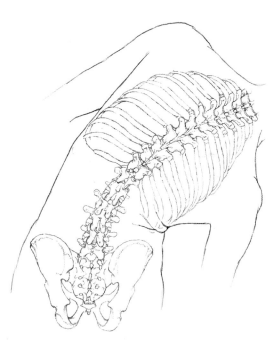

6.9 SIDE BENDING, LIMITED IN LUMBAR REGION

SPINAL CONDITIONS

Scoliosis. Scoliosis is a lateral curvature of the spinal column. It most often begins in the thoracic region but has implications for the cervical and lumbar regions. There are two types. A structural scoliosis is created by a difference in the height of the vertebral bodies. For some unknown reason, one side of the vertebral body grows higher than the other. This is called an idiopathic scoliosis, from the Greek meaning "unknown disease." Structural scoliosis is usually noticed during the growth spurts of the first year of life, at around six or seven years, and again at puberty. If you notice a young student with what you think is scoliosis, notify her parent immediately, so she can get proper care. In very severe cases, the lateral curvature—and thus accompanying side bending—can impinge on the healthy functioning of the lungs and other organs. Before the discovery of antibiotics, people suffering from severe scoliosis would occasionally die from pneumonia due to decreased lung capacity.

The second type of scoliosis is a lateral curvature of the vertebral column caused by the way the body is habitually used—always rotating in one direction at work, for example, or always carrying something heavy on one shoulder. This functional scoliosis is created by changes in soft tissue, like muscles, rather than by the uneven growth of bone.

There is a simple way to tell the difference between a structural and a functional scoliosis. Have your student stand in Tadasana and then bend forward. She should not try to stretch out in Uttanasana but rather just hang forward. Now stand behind her and observe her back. If she has a functional scoliosis, the stretch will result in the soft tissue releasing, and her back will look even from side to side. If she has a structural scoliosis, it will be more apparent that one side of her rib cage is higher than the other.

Understanding the law of side bending and rotation will allow you to make a very accurate guess as to which way your student's scoliosis exists. Stand behind her and, after asking her permission, place your hands around her mid-rib cage, using the space between your thumb and index finger to lightly hold the cage.

Now notice the difference in the thickness of her cage from front to back. If she has a right thoracic scoliosis, you will feel that her rib cage is a little thicker on the right, as it has rotated backward. This means that she is rotated right. According to the law, she is therefore side bent left. Since a scoliosis is named for its convexity (in this case her right side) and the student is side bent left, this would be a right thoracic scoliosis. This is the most common form of thoracic scoliosis.

If the student has a right thoracic scoliosis, her cervical and lumbar spines will side bend in the opposite directions in order to compensate for the shift. To imagine this, stand up and side bend your thoracic spine to the left, simulating a right thoracic scoliosis. Notice how your weight shifts to your right foot and your head tilts left.

The body will compensate for this shift. In order to keep both of your feet evenly on the ground and to tilt your head so that your eyes remain parallel to the floor, your body will side bend your cervical and lumbar curves, so that they are now side bending back to the right, the opposite direction from the primary thoracic curve. This will allow both feet to touch the floor evenly and the head to be straight. These compensatory side bends in the cervical and lumbar regions are attempts by the body to stand vertically in the face of the primary scoliosis.

However, in a right thoracic scoliosis, not only will there be three side bending actions, there will be rotational ones as well. Remember that side bending and rotation occur together in the vertebral column. Therefore in a right thoracic scoliosis the following conditions will exist:

Spinal Region	Side Bend	Rotation
cervical spine	right	right, except for C1
thoracic spine*	left	right
lumbar spine	right	left

*primary curve of a right thoracic scoliosis

Asana for Scoliosis. Because of this complicated picture of rotations and side bending, I advise that unless you know otherwise, since a right thoracic scoliosis is the most common type, you begin as if the thoracic spine is the primary scoliosis. Suggest movements that help the thoracic scoliosis and secondarily the cervical and lumbar segments. Obviously some of the movements you choose to help the thoracic area will be counter to the cervical and lumbar areas, but proceed anyway.

Since every structural scoliosis has a functional overlay, stretching the soft tissue of the back and trunk can help a student with scoliosis, regardless of whether it is structural and functional together or just functional.

The key to helping scoliosis is to stretch the concavity, strengthen the convexity, and derotate the rotated segments. These are the principles that will help you help your student. Here are some simple stretches that you may find effective.

▶ Standing: In Tadasana, have the student stand with one foot slightly forward of the other to help derotate the spine. For example, in a right thoracic scoliosis, try having him put his left foot slightly forward to increase weight-bearing on it and thus help to reduce the side bending in that area.

▶ Sitting: Observe the student sitting. He may actually sit more evenly if he sits a little bit forward with one side of his pelvis. When he is sitting asymmetrically, check the level of the pelvic rim to make sure that it is even. Be sure to ask permission to touch him first.

▶ Hanging: Encourage the student to hang whenever possible. He can hang from his hands or knees from playground equipment or from his pelvis in a pelvic sling.

▶ Ardha Adho Mukha Svanasana and Adho Mukha Svanasana: Have the student practice Ardha Adho Mukha Svanasana with her hands on the wall and her trunk at 90 degrees to the floor. Once in the position, she can move her feet to one side and/or drop one hand a little lower until her spine evens out. When she practices Adho Mukha Svanasana on a nonskid mat, it may even out her spine if she experiments with moving either one hand forward or one foot back or both. Remember, scoliosis is an asymmetrical problem, so asymmetry is often what is needed to help it.

▶ Adho Mukha Virasana: This pose can be very helpful. After the student bends forward in Adho Mukha Virasana, have him walk his arms forward on the floor. When he has done this, have him walk his arms to the side that causes the concavity of the curve to stretch out. Hold the pose for 10 breaths.

▶ Side-Lying with Blocking: Wedging props under a part of the body when a person is lying supine is

called blocking. Determine which way the student is curved. Set up a nonskid mat for her to lie on. Add a blanket on top for comfort, if desired. Then have her lie down on her side, so that the convexity is down, over a rolled towel or rolled small blanket. This will reverse the curve by reversing the side bending. Add other padding to support her head, neck, and legs, as necessary. She can lie for as long as 10 minutes.

▶ Savasana with Blocking: This is a little tricky but worth it. Have the student lie on a nonskid mat for Savasana, with no other props. Now determine by looking which shoulder is high, and support it with a rolled towel. Place another rolled towel under the back of his lower ribs on the side that is the lowest, using the towel as a wedge. You can use a towel as a wedge under the opposite buttock. After you place the towel, ask for his permission to check if the anterior superior iliac spines (ASISs) are even. If they are not, adjust the towel under the buttocks. Finally, add support to the head and neck, a large roll to the back of the knees, and a smaller one to the back of the Achilles tendon. Cover his eyes with a soft cloth and his body with a blanket, and let him rest for 20 minutes.

Sciatica. This is the irritation of the sciatic nerve. It usually has one of two causes. The first is discogenic (caused by the disc), which means that the intervertebral disc has moved out of place and is placing pressure on all or part of the nerve. When this pressure occurs, the student may feel numbness, tingling, and/or radiating pain down the leg. The more distally the symptoms are felt, the more severe the compression. If the student has neurological signs like this, she should consult a health care professional. If her symptoms include bowel or bladder problems, she should seek immediate aid. If you think that she has discogenic sciatica, refer her to a health care professional for positive diagnosis and then to a very experienced yoga teacher for help.

The second cause of sciatica may be piriformis syndrome. This form of sciatica is caused by pressure on the sciatic nerve as is passes under or between one of the external rotators in the hip, the piriformis muscle. Stretching the rotator muscles can help this problem. See the Experiential Anatomy section in chapter 8 for instructions on how to practice a stretch for the external rotators of the hip that may help lessen or prevent piriformis syndrome.

EXPERIENTIAL ANATOMY

For Practicing

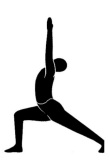

6.10

VIRABHA-

DRASANA I

Applied Practice: Virabhadrasana I

Prop: 1 nonskid mat

Take Care: To protect your front knee when it is bent, make sure the knee points over your little toe and is held at 90 degrees of flexion.

ONE OF THE MOST common beliefs many yoga students have is that the lumbar spine should be flattened or lengthened in all poses except back bends. When you practice standing poses, are you attempting to flatten your lumbar spine? Students often struggle with Virabhadrasana I and never really enjoy it because they are trying to flex the lumbar spine.

Take the starting position for Virabhadrasana I on your nonskid mat (Figure 6.10). Facing your right leg with your arms lifted overhead, bend your knee and allow your lumbar spine to arch naturally. Do not try to tuck the tailbone. In fact, do the exact opposite: allow the lumbar to arch and the tailbone to lift slightly. Encourage your breastbone to lift as well. Place your arms in front of your face, reaching up strongly with your arms and pressing your palms together. If your neck will allow, drop your head back, part your lips, and soften your eyes. Remember to keep your breath moving and soft.

Feel how arched your back is. Lean your weight backward onto your straight back leg. This pose is actually a back bend, and when practiced that way, it will feel dynamic and satisfying. Inhale as you come up, and practice to the other side.

For Teaching

6.11

MARICHY-

ASANA III

Applied Teaching: Marichyasana III

Props: 1 chair • 1 nonskid mat

Take Care: In order to protect the lower back, make sure that students twist the pelvis with the whole spine in Marichyasana III and do not hold it stationary so that the spine and pelvis move together.

TRY THIS YOURSELF first and then have the student do it. Sit on the forward edge of a stable simple chair, with your feet flat on the floor. Now let your lumbar flex, rounding out toward the back of the chair. Try to twist to the right, and note the difficulty. Now come back to facing forward once again in your sitting posture, and create a normal lordosis. Now twist in the same direction, and notice the difference.

Ask your student to sit on a nonskid mat. When he bends his right knee to his chest in preparation to practice Marichyasana III, he brings his lumbar spine into flexion, especially the side of the lumbar where the knee is bent (Figure 6.11). Remember that the lumbar has a minimal ability to rotate, due to facet direction. Trying to twist the lumbar during flexion makes rotation even more difficult.

To improve the student's pose, have him focus on lifting upward, so his lumbar spine comes closer to the normal lumbar lordosis. He can do this by shifting his weight off his left buttock and mainly onto his right buttock. This action will help him elongate the spine upward, bringing more of a normal curve to the lumbar spine, thus improving his ability to twist.

LINKS

Awareness practice: observe the effects that different chairs have on the curve of your lumbar spine. If you spend some time at this, you will find that most chairs do not enhance the normal lumbar curve and, in fact, actually cause you to sit in too much lumbar flexion. An interesting book on this topic is *The Chair: Rethinking Culture, Body, and Design* by Galen Cranz (New York: W. W. Norton, 2000). For a comprehensive yoga program for back and neck pain relief, consult *Back Care Basics* by Mary Pullig Schatz, M.D. (Berkeley, CA: Rodmell Press, 1992).

The Sacrum 7

THE PYRAMID-SHAPED SACRUM is the site where the vertebral column (sacrum) and pelvic girdle (ilium) intersect. This is the site of union between the upper and lower body, and it functions as a large part of the posterior wall of the pelvis. The sacroiliac joint is a frequent site of problems for practitioners of asana. This chapter explains why.

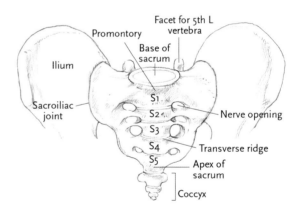

7.1 ANTERIOR SACROILIAC JOINT

BONES

The sacrum is created by the fusion of five vertebrae (Figure 7.1; see the sagittal view at Figure 3.1). This fusion is not complete until after the twenty-fifth year of life. The degree of curve of the sacrum bone is about the same as that of a saucer, with the concavity facing anteriorly.

The superior sacrum, sometimes called the base of the sacrum, has two oval superior facet surfaces that articulate with the fifth lumbar vertebra facets. These sacral facet surfaces face posteriorly and

oppose the lumbar facets, which face anteriorly.

The anterior surface of S1, called the sacral promontory, protrudes into the pelvic cavity. One can note as well the existence of transverse ridges on the anterior sacrum, which identify where the five vertebrae were fused together. On the posterior surface of the sacrum are a series of ridges that run vertically. These are called the middle

81

sacral crest, which has tubercles—the intermediate crests and the lateral crests—that are like primitive spinous processes. Lateral to the intermediate crest are openings for the passage of nerves.

At the distal end of the sacrum, which is called the apex, is the coccyx bone. It is made up of three to five bones that are fused together. This bone serves as the site of muscle and ligament attachment.

JOINTS

It would seem that something as concrete as a joint in the human body could not be controversial. However, there has been debate about whether the sacroiliac joint moves at all and, if so, how much. But as many yoga students can testify, this joint definitely moves. Furthermore, yoga students know that if the sacroiliac joint if is not moving according to anatomical principles (discussed later in this chapter), it can cause discomfort not only during asana practice but also during the activities of daily life.

The sacroiliac joint (SI joint) consists of the union of the convex surface of the sacrum and the concave surface of the ilium. Both joint surfaces are covered with a thin plate of cartilage. In later life, the space of the joint is filled with synovial fluid and thus acts as a gliding joint. The joint surfaces join such that the sacrum is at a diagonal angle of approximately 30 degrees from the vertical, with the promontory anterior and coccyx posterior. The neutral position of the sacrum in standing is *not* vertical. When your student stands with her sacrum vertical, she is not standing in the neutral position for the sacroiliac joint.

The most important thing to remember about the sacroiliac joint is that its major function is stability. There is definitely some movement needed at the sacroiliac joint, but it is quite minimal. When this stability is disturbed, and the bones are no longer in their neutral position but are separating slightly, the lig-

aments around the joint are stressed, and discomfort or pain can result.

To help create this stability, the sacroiliac joint surfaces are shaped to facilitate the wedging of the sacrum down into the ilia of the pelvis during weight bearing. When standing, the incumbent weight of the trunk forces the sacrum into the pelvis. This pressing down of the sacrum helps to create stability at the joint by keeping the ilia and sacrum in close proximity. This is called a self-locking mechanism.

Thus stability in the joint is greatest when standing. An unlocking motion occurs when one sits down. This occurs in part because the abdominal muscles are less active as support during sitting, and the sacrum is not wedged as firmly down in the pelvis as during standing.

There are significant gender differences in the structure of the SI joint that contribute to a greater instability in the joint for women. These differences are related to the need for an obstetric pelvis in women. The first structural difference is that the female joint generally has a smaller and flatter surface for joint articulation. Second, the female joint often articulates at only two segments with the pelvis, instead of at three for the male. This lesser degree of congruence at the joint surfaces decreases stability. Additionally the female sacral ligaments are subject to softening during the hormonal changes that accompany menstruation, pregnancy, and lactation. Finally there is additional strain on the female sacroiliac joint during walking. Here is how the strain happens.

The female acetabula are wider apart than the male acetabula in a proportional body. The wider the acetabula are apart, the greater the torque across the sacroiliac joint during each step of walking. To visualize this, hold a towel in front of you with your hands wide apart. Now move one hand forward, as if your hand were your acetabulum in walking. Note the torquing and twisting throughout the length of the towel. Now move your hands

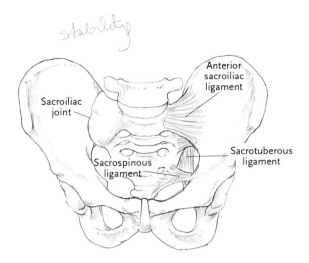

stability

7.2 ANTERIOR SACROILIAC JOINT, WITH ANTERIOR LIGAMENTS ON ONE SIDE

7.3 POSTERIOR SACROILIAC JOINT, WITH POSTERIOR LIGAMENTS ON ONE SIDE

closer together; when you "walk" this time, there will be less torque. This is exactly what happens in the female pelvis: each step has a greater chance of stress across the SI joint. All of these factors contribute to the more frequent dysfunction of the sacroiliac joint in females.

CONNECTIVE TISSUE

The function of the sacral ligaments, like all other ligaments in the body, is to provide support for joints. It is especially important that the sacroiliac ligaments are not overstretched in the practice of asana. Once these ligaments are overstretched, not only do they no longer provide the support necessary, but the overstretched ligaments never go back to their previous state. Remember that the main function of the sacroiliac joint is one of stability, not mobility.

Three ligaments support the sacroiliac joint:

▸ The anterior sacroiliac ligament connects the anterior sacrum to the medial ilium. It is broad and flat and is stretched on external rotation of the hip joint (Figure 7.2).

▸ The posterior sacroiliac ligament is one of the strongest of the area. One part runs from the dor-

sum of the sacrum to the tuberosity of the ilium; the other part runs obliquely from the third tubercle of the posterior sacrum to the posterior superior spine of the ilium (Figure 7.3).

▸ The interosseous sacroiliac ligament connects the tuberosity of the sacrum and the ilium.

These ligaments connect the sacrum and ischium:

▸ The sacrotuberous ligament connects the posterior inferior spine of the ilium, the lateral margin of the sacrum, and the coccyx and the tuberosity of the ischium.

▸ The sacrospinous ligament connects the lateral sacrum and coccyx to the spine of the ischium.

NERVES

The sacral plexus is formed by nerve roots from the lumbar, sacral, and coccygeal areas. The first of these nerves is L4 and the last is C1. The L4-S3 nerves converge and exit the pelvis as the sciatic nerve. For more details about the sacral plexus, see chapter 6.

Muscles

One of best ways to create stability in a joint is to strengthen the muscles that cross that joint. Unfortunately, there is only one muscle that crosses the sacroiliac joint, the piriformis. While it is technically considered a muscle of the hip joint, it is included here because of its effect on the sacroiliac.

The piriformis originates from the anterior sacrum, between the first four sacral foramina, and it inserts into the top of the greater trochanter. The muscle lies almost horizontal. When it contracts, it acts as an external rotator of the hip and aids in adduction and extension. Additionally it can help to stabilize the pelvis during walking.

Remember that the sciatic nerve passes under the piriformis, or is sometimes intertwined in it, on its way to exit the pelvis. Therefore a tight piriformis muscle can press on the nerve. This pressure can cause pain along the path of the sciatic nerve—sciatica—which is called piriformis syndrome. See chapter 8 for a stretch for this muscle.

Kinesiology

Mechanics of the Sacroiliac Joint. The entire vertebral column is balanced on the sacrum. In fact, the crucial mechanical joint of the spine is L5–S1. Due to the opposite curves of the lumbar spine and the sacrum, there is an increased shearing stress at the lumbo-sacral angle. This is the shearing stress of the incumbent weight of the column pushing anteriorly, due to the angle of L5 as it joins S1.

The facets of L5–S1 are in a weight-bearing position. When standing, L5 would move forward on S1 due to gravity except for the angle of the facets, as detailed in the Bones section of this chapter. The angle of the L5 and S1 facets create a braking effect on the vertebral bodies to keep L5 from sliding forward on S1. This can contribute to a compression of the articular synovial linings at this level.

While the primary function of the sacroiliac joint is stability, some passive joint movements occur there. The first of these movements is nutation, from the Latin *nutare,* meaning "to nod" (Figure 7.4). Nutation refers to the movement of S1 in relationship to the lumbar spine and the pelvis; it is the anterior movement of S1 that accompanies lumbar extension. This means that when you back bend your lumbar spine, your S1 vertebra passively moves anteriorly. The opposite movement is counternutation, which is the passive movement of S1 posteriorly, when you perform flexion of your lumbar spine (Figure 7.5).

It is important to understand the relationship of the movements of the lumbar spine and the sacrum. When you perform a back bend—perform active spinal extension—your sacrum *passively* nutates, and S1 moves anteriorly. When you forward bend—perform active spinal flexion—your sacrum passively counternutates, and S1 moves posteriorly. Nutation and counternutation are passive movements only but they *must* accompany extension and flexion, respectively, for them to be normal, healthy, and complete.

These movements of extension with nutation and flexion with counternutation are called the lumbo-sacral rhythm. To experience this, stand near a chair and put your hand over your sacrum, which is located just below your waist and is hard and curved outward. Now sit down slowly, and notice how your S1 counternutates as you sit. In other words, your S1 moves posteriorly at exactly the same time that your lumbar spine flexes. Once you have sat down, notice that S1 will move back to its more neutral and slightly nutated position if you sit with your spine long and lifted, with neutral spinal curves.

To complete the experiment, keep your hand on your sacrum and stand up. You will notice the rhythm in reverse. As you begin to stand, your sacrum will nutate as you lean forward and then move slightly back toward counternutation as you come to a neutral standing position. This is nor-

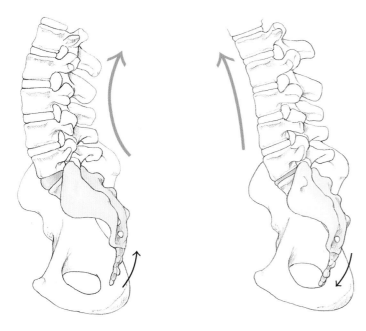

7.4 (FAR LEFT) NUTATION

7.5 (LEFT) COUNTERNUTATION

mal lumbo-sacral rhythm. If you have some form of sacroiliac dysfunction, this rhythm will be disrupted. It is sometimes possible to guess the cause of a student's back pain: students with discogenic lower back pain will usually prefer standing to sitting, because sitting increases the pressure on the disc. But students with sacroiliac dysfunction will usually have the most trouble during the transitional movements, from sitting to standing, and vice versa.

Sacroiliac and Iliosacral Dysfunctions. The way to avoid creating dysfunction at the sacroiliac joint is to move in such a way that the sacrum and pelvis always move together. This is true for all asana movements, especially twists and forward bends.

There are two major dysfunctions at the sacroiliac joint. One is the movement of the sacrum in relationship to the ilium, called sacroiliac dysfunction. The second is iliosacral dysfunction, which is the displacement of the ilium in relationship to the sacrum.

Please understand that these are relative terms; nevertheless there is a difference in the two dysfunctions. Sacroiliac dysfunction is related to the spine itself being stuck at the sacrum level in relationship to the pelvis. Iliosacral dysfunction is the pelvis moving in relationship to the sacrum and is more affected by the muscles of the legs and pelvis pulling on one of the ilia. One of the causes of these dysfunctions can be postural habits, which are almost always asymmetrical for the pelvis, either standing, sitting, or sleeping postures.

Sacroiliac dysfunction specifically is a rotation of the sacrum in relationship to the ilium. This is more related to how the spine is used in relationship to the ilium. Once again, sacroiliac dysfunction can be created by asymmetrical postural habits, in this case of the sacrum. Both of these dysfunctions can be created by the way certain asana are performed, especially twists of all kinds and seated forward bends. When you move your spine in a twisting motion, for example, while keeping your pelvis fixed and still, you are creating a stress at the SI joint and can create sacroiliac dysfunction.

Iliosacral dysfunction is either an anterior or posterior positional fault of the ilium in relationship to the sacrum. Thus the ilium can be rotated and stuck either anteriorly or posteriorly in relationship to the sacrum. An anterior rotation is called anterior torsion, and a posterior rotation is called posterior torsion (Figures 7.6 and 7.7). Remember, the term *torsion* refers specifically to the movement of the ilium in relationship to the sacrum. This usually happens on one side or the other. Because the acetabulum is on the lateral side of each ilium, by the movement of the acetabulum either anteriorly or posteriorly, a torsion can affect the placement of the femur.

If a student complains of a short leg on the right, for example, three different things could be causing it. First, she could actually have an anatomically short leg, which is the least common reason. The next reason could be that she has a posterior torsion on the right side. Remember, this means that her right ilium is rotated posteriorly. As it rotates posteriorly, it draws the acetabulum posteriorly as well, in effect shortening the right leg. The third reason that her right leg could appear short is that the left ilium is rotated anteriorly. In this case, technically she would not have a short leg but rather a long leg, because she has an anterior torsion right, making her left leg appear longer than her right one.

If you ascertain that the short leg is created by the second reason, that is, a torsion of the ilium, you can have her twist in such a way as to bring her ilum back into place. For example, if she has a left posterior torsion, have her twist for twice as long to the right as to the left in a pose like Marichyasana III, thus encouraging her left pelvis to rotate forward.

7.6 (RIGHT) ANTERIOR TORSION OF THE ILIUM

7.7 (FAR RIGHT) POSTERIOR TORSION OF THE ILIUM

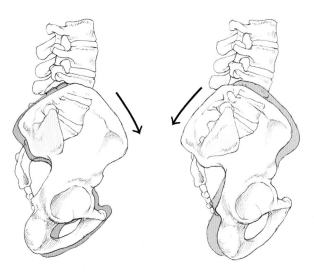

Experiential Anatomy

For Practicing

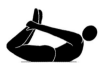

7.8

DHANURASANA

Applied Practice 1: Dhanurasana

Props: 1 nonskid mat • 1 blanket

Take Care: Do not practice these poses while pregnant, or when diagnosed disc disease, spondylosis, or spondylolisthesis is present.

BEGIN BY LOCATING your sacrum with your hand. When you are ready for back bends in your practice, fold your blanket in half and then in half again, and place it on your mat. Lie on your belly (unless you are pregnant). Take a moment to place your hand over your sacrum again, to be sure of its location.

Stretch out first one leg and then the other to lengthen the abdomen and upper thigh area. Bend your knees one by one and clasp the ankles. With an exhalation, lift up into Dhanurasana (Figure 7.8). Pay attention to what happens to the sacrum as you do this. It will be nutating S1 down toward the mat as your lumbar spine extends. Hold for a few breaths and come down, resting a moment before repeating.

This time, focus your attention on the S1 vertebra. Reach back and place your fingers on S1 to remind yourself exactly where it is in your body. Now, as you exhale and lift up into the pose again, consciously press S1 to the floor and imagine that everything else is lifting upward. With this thought, you are consciously facilitating nutation. Remember, nutation must accompany extension if extension is to be healthy. Try this pose one more time, again focusing on nutation.

When done, rest for a few cycles of breath and proceed to Practice 2.

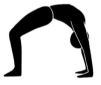

7.9

URDHVA
DHANURASANA

Applied Practice 2: Urdhva Dhanurasana

Prop: 1 nonskid mat

Take Care: Do not practice these poses while pregnant, or when diagnosed disc disease, spondylosis, or spondylolisthesis is present.

AS YOU ARE READY, turn over and lie on your back for Urdhva Dhanurasana (Figure 7.9). Place your feet near your buttocks, with your toes turned inward; place your hands directly beneath the socket of the shoulder joint, with your fingers turned outward. Exhale, and bring your lower back to the floor so you are in flexion and counternutation. With the next exhalation, move your pelvis out and up and over your feet, in a strong and fairly quick movement. Be sure to lead with your tailbone to stretch out, as if moving the tailbone along the inner thighs.

In the first part of coming up into Urdhva Dhanurasana, you will be keeping your spine in flexion, but this will change about halfway up. Pay attention as you go up to the exact point where the lumbar spine begins to extend and your sacrum begins to nutate. As you straighten your arms and legs, consciously lift the pose, but not from the coccyx. If you lift from your coccyx, that would be counternutation and the opposite of the nutation needed for extension. Rather, lift from S1 to facilitate nutation, so your coccyx actually goes down in relationship to your S1 vertebra.

Many yoga students are taught to lift from the tailbone in this pose, but that is kinesiologically illogical. Extension and nutation go together as natural movements in your body. If you want to facilitate extension, you need to nutate as you lift into the last half of the pose.

Hold the pose for several breaths and keep lifting from your S1 vertebra. Visualize connection between your coccyx and your heels as they both move down. Make sure your feet stay parallel and your inner thighs rotate inward and downward. Come down, rest, breathe, and repeat before moving to the next pose in your practice.

For Teaching

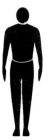

7.10
TADASANA

Applied Teaching 1: The SI Joint in Tadasana
Prop: 1 nonskid mat
Take Care: Stand on an even surface.
HAVE YOUR STUDENT stand on his mat in Tadasana (Figure 7.10), and walk all the way around him, observing his pelvic and sacral positions. Remember that a neutral sacrum is diagonal and not vertical.

After asking permission to touch, first place your flat hands on his iliac crests to ascertain if they are level with the floor. The crests are, of course, curved bones, and so your hands will not be resting on completely flat surfaces. Rather, try to imagine a line tangential to the highest point of the crest and guess whether that line is parallel to the floor. Do not be discouraged if this is not easy to discover at first; just keep practicing it with your students or willing family members. This position is the neutral position of the pelvis.

Once you find the neutral position of his pelvis, begin to note the angle of the sacrum. It should be diagonal and not vertical. If the sacrum is vertical, it has become unlocked from the ilia, and this creates a less stable relationship at the bottom of the column. In order to lock the sacrum into the ilia, the student needs to stand with his sacrum in that 30-degree diagonal line; when he does so, the tops of his ilia will be parallel to the floor as well. Note: this is *not* a movement created by tucking the tailbone, which is sometimes recommended.

7.11
JANU
SIRSASANA

Applied Teaching 2: The SI Joint in Janu Sirsasana
Prop: 1 nonskid mat • 1 towel
Take Care: Do not practice this pose if it causes pain in your sacroiliac area.
HAVE YOUR STUDENT practice the seated forward bend, Janu Sirsasana (Figure 7.11). Ask her permission to touch her. Then kneel behind her and feel her ilia and her sacroiliac joint. This pose is an asymmetrical one and therefore can cause torque at the sacroiliac joint. Make sure that she rolls forward into the forward bend, especially from the ilia of the bent knee side. In other words, have her create the forward bend not by bending over

her straight leg but rather by reaching and bending forward from the bent knee side ilium, thus reducing the torque over her SI joint.

Many students stretch forward from the spine of the bent knee side, but this tends to separate the vertebral column/sacrum from the pelvis, which is left behind by this focus. Instead, make sure your student bends forward from the pelvis itself around the concavity of the femoral head to move the ilium, sacrum, and column together. To add some extra help, wedge the edge of a folded towel under the upper, outer area of the back thigh of the bent leg.

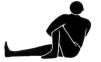

7.12
MARICHY-
ASANA III

Applied Teaching 3: The SI Joint in Marichyasana III
Prop: 1 nonskid mat
Take Care: Do not practice this pose if it causes pain in your sacroiliac area.

WHEN YOUR STUDENT practices Marichyasana III, make sure that he begins the twist from his pelvis (Figure 7.12). In other words, make sure that he moves his straight leg forward on the floor, so that the hip socket of the straight leg is several inches, maybe even as many as 6 inches, ahead of the hip socket of the bent knee. This action will create the twist at the very base of the pose. Do not allow him to keep his acetabula even. This will cause the twist to come at the SI joint, thus separating or straining the SI joint. Instead, make sure he moves his straight leg forward, thus beginning the twist from the pelvis, not the sacrum.

If he begins the pose by anchoring his pelvis before twisting, he will in effect be pulling his spine and sacroiliac joint into the twist, while turning his pelvis back in the other direction. Remember, when the sacrum and ilia move in separate directions, this is the definition of sacroiliac dysfunction. Be sure that the student moves his pelvis as the basis of this and all twists.

LINK

While it may seem counterintuitive, those suffering with persistent posterior torsion of the ilia often feel relief when they wear shoes with a slight heel. Suggest to students with posterior torsion that they experiment with wearing shoes with heels one to one and a half inches high instead of flat shoes. (Men can wear boots.) This slight lift can help to create a lumbar curve. This curve will help to rotate the posterior ilium anteriorly, thus bringing it into a more normal position.

PART THREE:

The Lower Extremity

The Pelvis, Hip Joint, and Femur 8

EVERY MAN IS A BUILDER OF A TEMPLE CALLED HIS BODY.

—HENRY DAVID THOREAU

IN THE FIRST yoga class I took with B. K. S. Iyengar, he began by teaching us Tadasana. What was so exciting was the way he integrated the philosophy of yoga into the actions of the body as he instructed the pose. He spoke of how the feet were *bhakti* yogis, that they served us by supporting us selflessly all day long. He pointed out that the thighs were *karma* yogis, that they did the work of walking. Throughout the class he clarified the actions and power of the lower extremities in asana by emphasizing the standing poses. Since then I have had a deeper appreciation for the importance of the legs and feet and their contribution to our practice.

The word *pelvis* means "basin," which is exactly what the pelvis is: a basin to hold the organs of digestion, assimilation, elimination, and reproduction. The pelvis is also the pot out of which the spine grows; thus the position of the pelvis is critical for creating spinal alignment and health. The pelvis joins with the vertebral column through the sacrum and simultaneously balances itself through the hip joints, thus becoming a central fulcrum for the movements of asana.

To the yoga practitioner, in addition to its anatomical significance, the pelvis is the site of the lower three *chakras*, spiritual wheels that fuel the arising of kundalini energy and contribute to spiritual evolution. It is said that *apana,* the feminine energy living in all people regardless of gender, has its home in the pelvis. The pelvic floor is important too, as it is not only the site of important muscles that help to support the organs of the pelvis but also where aspirants focus techniques, such as Mulabandha (Root Lock), to control the movement of their energy.

The hip joint is important for so many asana that understanding its movements and limitations is key to teaching standing poses and forward bends, in particular.

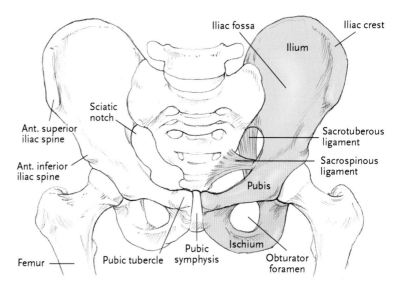

8.1 ANTERIOR PELVIS,
WITH THE ANTERIOR HIP LIGAMENTS

BONES

The pelvis is made up of three bones, the largest of which is the ilium, which forms the broad, flat bone of the pelvis. On the medial side of the ilia is a fossa known as the iliac fossa, where the iliacus muscle originates. The top of the ilia is called the iliac crest; it can be felt at the lower side waist (Figure 8.1).

The ability to locate the bony landmarks on the pelvis, both visually and tactilely, can make helping your student easier. Two important bony landmarks are found on the ilia. In the front of the body is the knobby anterior superior iliac crest. You can feel this at the lateral side of the low abdomen; sometimes when you lie on your belly it will poke the floor. The other landmark is the posterior superior iliac crest. It is found just over the sacroiliac joint on the posterior side of the body. Below each of these prominences is found a smaller crest, the anterior and the posterior inferior iliac crest, respectively (Figure 8.2).

The ischium makes up one-third of the pelvis and provides the two, rounded, firm ends of the pelvis on which we sit, the ischial tuberosities. Another important bony landmark on the ischium is the greater sciatic notch, made up in part of the ischium and the ilia. The greater sciatic notch is the passageway for the sciatic nerve to exit the pelvis. Distal to the greater sciatic notch is the lesser sciatic notch. This latter notch is converted into a true foramen by the sacrotuberous and sacrospinous ligaments; it allows for the passage of the tendon of the obturator internus muscle as well as nerves and blood vessels. The greater sciatic notch provides the opening for the passage of the sciatic nerve as well as for the piriformis muscle.

The third bone of the pelvis is the pubic bone, which also makes up one-third of the pelvis. The two rami (arms) of the pubis join with the ischium. On the anterior portion of the pubic bone is the pubic tubercle, a prominence that serves as the attachment for muscles. A rami of the pubic bone and a rami of the ischium join to create the obturator foramen. The obturator vessels and nerves exit the pelvis through this opening.

The front lower wall of the pelvis is created by the pubic symphysis, which is the union of the left and right anterior pubic rami. The pubic symphysis is composed of strong ligaments which hold the pubic rami together but which soften during pregnancy due to hormones and which separate

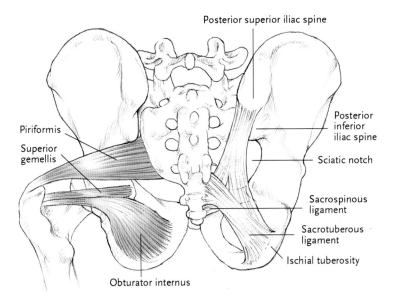

Posterior superior iliac spine

Piriformis

Superior
gemellis

Posterior
inferior
iliac spine

Sciatic notch

Sacrospinous
ligament

Sacrotuberous
ligament

Ischial tuberosity

Obturator internus

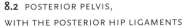

8.2 POSTERIOR PELVIS,
WITH THE POSTERIOR HIP LIGAMENTS

slightly to allow for the passage of the baby from the pelvis.

There are two ways to classify the opening in the central pelvis. The greater or false pelvis is the opening made up of the most superior aspects of the pelvis and is, of course, open on the anterior side. The lesser or true pelvis is the deeper cavity and is bounded by bony walls. The inlet of the lesser pelvis allows for the baby's head to drop during the last part of pregnancy or during the early stages of labor. The pelvic outlet is the bony opening for the birth of the baby and is bounded in part by the pubic symphysis and the rami of the pubic bones, the sacrum, the coccyx, the inner ischium, and the lower inner ilium.

Gender Differences in the Pelvis. The male and female pelvis differ in a number of ways. These can be seen in the fetus as early as the fourth month. The differences are of course related to obstetric considerations. The female pelvis is more delicate, the ilia flare out more, and the acetabula and ischial tuberosities are farther apart. The superior inlet of the female pelvis is rounder, the cavity of the pelvis is shallower and wider, and the sacrum is wider and shorter. The coccyx is more movable. The acetabula are smaller and project more ante-

riorly, and the pubic symphysis is less deep. One interesting fact about the pelvis is that its size, unlike other bones, is not necessarily influenced by the size of the individual skeleton. In other words, even in tall people, the pelvis is not necessarily proportionally bigger.

Femur. The femur is the largest, longest, and strongest single bone in the body. It has a slight anterior curve that improves its ability to bear weight. The head of the femur presents a full rounded surface, which forms one half of the hip joint where it joins with the acetabulum (see the Joints section in this chapter).

The head of the femur tapers into a thin neck, which is the most vulnerable part of the upper femur. This is the most common site of fracture from falls in the elderly. Fractures happen to women more frequently due to the increased occurrence of osteoporosis at this site. In fact, some physical therapists believe that a spontaneous fracture of the femoral neck occurs first, resulting in a subsequent fall.

The neck of the femur has an angle of about 125 degrees to the shaft of the femur. The greater trochanter is a projection to be found at the site where the neck and the body of the femur join. It serves as an attachment point for muscles. It is easy to find the greater trochanter on your body. Stand in Tadasana, and feel the lateral uppermost femur. The greater trochanter will be that bony knob projecting laterally and slightly anteriorly.

The lesser trochanter can be found on the posterior side of the femur, at the base of the neck. It is a major site for the insertion of the psoas major muscle, which cannot practically be palpated from the outside.

The intertrochanteric line runs in an oblique angle between the greater and lesser trochanters and serves as an attachment point for soft tissue.

The long shaft, or body, of the femur curves not only anteriorly but medially, to bring the distal femur underneath the hip joint proper. In women, because the acetabula tend to be wider apart, there tends to be more of a medial curve than in men. On the posterior surface of the shaft is a raised line that runs most of the length of the bone and is called the linea aspera. It provides a place for the attachment of various muscles of the hip joint.

The distal end of the femur forms two major prominences called the medial and lateral condyles. These form the superior surfaces of the knee joint and are joined together on the anterior surface and separated more distinctly on the posterior surface. (The knee joint is discussed in detail in chapter 9). The medial condyle is the larger; it projects a proximal prominence called the medial epicondyle, which serves as a site for the attachment of connective tissue, the medial collateral ligament of the knee. The lateral epicondyle is not as large as the medial one; it is the site of connection of the fibular collateral ligament of the knee joint.

Joints

One of the key joints of the pelvis is the sacroiliac joint, which is discussed in detail in chapter 7. The other key joint of the pelvis is the hip joint.

The hip joint is formed by the union of the head of the femur with the acetabulum (Figure 8.3). The acetabulum is a deep, circular joint formed by the fusing of the ilium, the ischium, and the pubic bone in the following proportions: two-fifths from the ilium and the ischium and one-fifth from the pubic bone. The pelvis proper and the acetabulum are completely fused by the twenty-fifth year of life.

The femur sits in the acetabulum at an angle that may at first seem counterintuitive. Many yoga teachers think of the head and neck of the femur joining at the hip joint in the frontal plane, but this is not so. There is an angle to this relationship called femoral anteversion. In other words, the neck of the femur points anteriorly about 10 to 25 degrees, using the frontal plane as the point of reference.

Another way to understand anteversion is to visualize observing your student as if you were over the top of her head, looking down on her like she was a column. Because of the normal position of anteversion of the femoral neck, you would clearly be able to see that her femoral heads are anterior to her hip sockets, not parallel to them.

This means that the greater trochanter is anterior of the actual hip joint (acetabulum and femoral head) when it is in the neutral position. If the student stands with her greater trochanter in the frontal plane, parallel with her hip socket, she is actually standing in external rotation. However, if this anteversion is more than about 30 degrees, she will probably demonstrate a lack of external rotation.

The opposite of anteversion is femoral retroversion. This occurs when the angle of the femoral neck and head as it enters the acetabulum is less than 10 degrees. In this case, the student will demonstrate an extreme limitation of internal rotation.

The position of most stability in the hip joint is not this neutral or Tadasana position. Instead, the position of most stability for the hip joint is when the femur is in slight abduction, flexion, and external rotation. You can experience this position for yourself. Stand up and imagine that you are going to pick up a heavy load. As you imagine yourself doing this, you will no doubt separate your feet, turn your feet slightly out, and bend your knees and flex your hips. This is the position that professional weightlifters use when lifting. It is also the position of stability created in such poses as Utthita Trikonasana and Ardha Chandrasana.

If you do the opposite—that is, internally rotate the femurs instead—you will move the head of your femurs out of their sockets slightly (adduction), thus reducing the congruence of the head of the femur and the acetabulum. In fact, after total hip replacement surgery, the doctor recommends that the patient not ever cross her legs with the involved leg on top. If she does so, sitting in flexion, adduction, and internal rotation with the involved leg, she will be moving the head of the femur out of the socket and into the position of dislocation. Remember that the angle the neck of the femur has in neutral is a slightly forward position, so it is easier than you might think to move the head of the femur away from the acetabulum.

CONNECTIVE TISSUE

The ligaments of the hip joint are some of the strongest in the body. As a whole, they tend to limit abduction. The first is the iliofemoral, which lies on the anterior surface of the joint and runs from the anterior femur, around the neck of the femur, to insert on the intertrochanteric line. This ligament is also called the Y ligament of Bigelow. This ligament can limit back bending asana if the student externally rotates and abducts her femurs. In back bending the ligament is stretched. If the student internally rotates during back bends, the ligament will be less stretched.

The pubofemoral ligament runs from the superior ramus of the pubis to the distal iliofemoral ligament. Finally the ischiofemoral ligament originates from the ischium and blends with the hip joint capsule to insert. All three of these ligaments serve to reinforce and support the hip capsule.

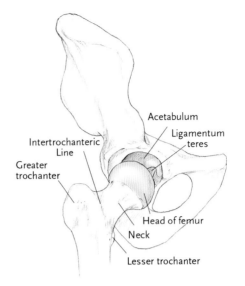

8.3 HEAD OF THE FEMUR IN ACETABULUM, WITH THE LIGAMENTUM TERES

The ligamentum teres has another special function, in addition to helping to hold the joint together. The head of the femur is nourished by a single blood vessel that passes through the acetabulum inside a ligament called the ligamentum teres. Because this blood vessel and ligament are somewhat delicate, injury to them can disrupt the blood supply to the femoral head and cause avascular necrosis of the femoral head.

The acetabulum has a fibrocartilaginous rim that creates a lip around the joint. Not only does this deepen the joint, but it also protects the bony rim of the acetabulum. The center of the socket itself is bone, but there is a ring of cartilage around the outer periphery of the acetabulum. This cartilage, as does all cartilage, protects bony surfaces and facilitates easy movement; it may be as much as 9 mm thick. A distinct difference has been found in the formation and thickness of this cartilage when comparing physically inactive cultures and those in which people are very physically active from a young age.

Another significant connective structure that affects the hip joint is the fascia lata. This fascial

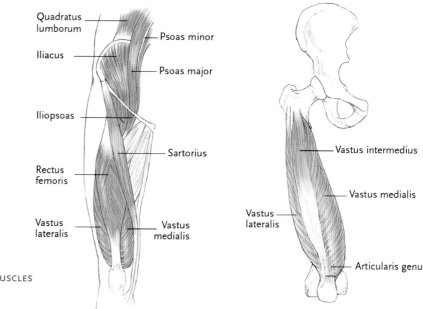

Quadratus
lumborum

Iliacus

Iliopsoas

Rectus
femoris

Vastus
lateralis

Psoas minor

Psoas major

Sartorius

Vastus
medialis

Vastus intermedius

Vastus medialis

Vastus
lateralis

Articularis genu

8.4 ANTERIOR ILIAC AND THIGH MUSCLES

sheath runs along the most lateral surface of the thigh; it arises from the pelvic bone, the thoracolumbar fascia, the inguinal ligament, and external abdominal fasciae. It travels down the outside of the thigh, connects with a variety of muscles, and finally inserts into multiple sites at the region of the distal femur.

Finally, over the area of the greater trochanter, the aponeurosis of the gluteus maximus muscle blends into the fascia lata and is called the iliotibial band.

NERVES

The nerves of the pelvic region originate from the lumbar and sacral nerve plexuses. They are discussed in detail in chapter 6.

MUSCLES

The muscles of the pelvis and thigh are some of the strongest and most important in the body. They anchor the spine to the pelvis and the pelvis to the femur, help to form the floor of the pelvis, and allow us to stand and locomote. The charts that follow will help you to learn about these muscles. They are grouped by location and muscle action.

Anterior iliac and thigh muscles: hip flexors and knee extensors. The muscles of the anterior thigh are some of the biggest in the body (Figures 8.4 and 8.5). They work together to initiate the first part of locomotion and to maintain the extension of the knee joint during walking and standing. Also known in part as the "quads," these muscles are strengthened by standing poses and are stretched by lunges and back bends

8.5 ANTERIOR ILIAC AND THIGH MUSCLES

MUSCLE	ORIGIN	INSERTION	ACTION
Psoas major	Transverse processes of all lumbar vertebrae; sides of T12–L5 vertebrae	Lesser trochanter	Flexes thigh and trunk; acting alone side bends trunk
Psoas minor	Sides of bodies of T12–L5 vertebrae	Lateral pubic bone	Flexes lumbar spine
Iliacus	Iliac fossa; iliac crest	With tendon of psoas major into lesser trochanter	Flexes the femur; flexes the trunk against gravity
Quadratus lumborum	Iliolumbar ligament and iliac crest	Inferior border of last rib and transverse process of first four lumbar vertebrae	Draws last rib toward pelvis or fixes it; side bends lumbar spine
Sartorius	ASIS	Medial superior tibial shaft	Flexes femur and rotates it laterally; flexes knee and then rotates it medially
Quadriceps femoris: rectus femoris (there are two heads of the rectus femoris)	ASIS for straight head; groove above acetabulum for reflected head	Quadriceps tendon at base of patella	Flexes hip joint; extends leg at knee joint
Quadriceps femoris: vastus lateralis	Posterior aspect of femur, from greater trochanter to lateral linea aspera of femur	Base and lateral patella; tendon of rectus femoris	Extends leg at knee joint
Quadriceps femoris: vastus medialis	Intertrochanteric line, medial linea aspera of femur	Medial border of patella	Extends leg at knee joint
Quadriceps femoris: vastus intermedius	Anterior and lateral surfaces of shaft of femur	Posterior surface of patella, forms part of quadriceps tendon, then inserts into tibial tuberosity	Extends leg at knee joint
Articularis genu	Anterior distal body of femur	Proximal synovial membrane of knee joint	Draws articular capsule proximally

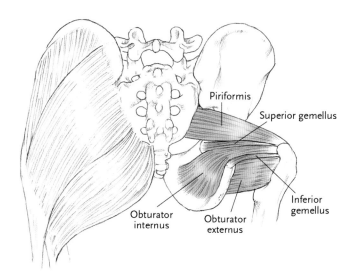

8.6 GLUTEAL MUSCLES

Gluteal muscles: hip extensors, abductors and external rotators. The muscles of the gluteal region are at the core of movements of the hip joint (Figures 8.6 and 8.7). They contribute to the poses that require strength and are absolutely necessary for standing on one leg. The piriformis, both obturators, and the gemelli are together called the external rotators. They are strengthened by standing poses, back bends, and balancing poses.

MUSCLE	ORIGIN	INSERTION	ACTION
Gluteus maximus	Posterior ilium, posterior lower sacrum, side of coccyx	Iliotibial band of fascia lata and gluteal tuberosity of femur	Extends and externally rotates femur
Gluteus medius	Lateral ilium	Greater trochanter	Abducts femur; anterior fibers rotate femur medially, posterior fibers rotate femur externally
Gluteus minimus	Lateral ilium and margin of greater sciatic notch	Greater trochanter	Abducts, medially rotates, and helps to flex femur
Tensor fasciae latae	Outer iliac crest, ASIS, and deep fascia lata	Iliotibial band at mid third of lateral femur	Flexes hip joint and helps to medially rotate it
Piriformis	Anterior surface of sacral segments 2, 3, and 4; sacrotuberous ligament; greater sciatic foramen	Greater trochanter	Rotates femur laterally; extends and abducts femur when thigh is flexed
Obturator internus	Internal rami of pubis and ischium	Medial greater trochanter	Rotates extended thigh laterally; abducts flexed thigh
Gemellus superior	Spine of ischium	Greater trochanter	Rotates extended thigh laterally; abducts flexed thigh
Gemellus inferior	Tuberosity of ischium	Greater trochanter	Rotates extended thigh laterally; abducts flexed thigh
Quadratus femoris	Lateral ischium	Posterior greater trochanter	Rotates extended thigh laterally; abducts flexed thigh
Obturator externus	External surface of obturator membrane; medial obturator foramen; rami of pubis and ischium	Medial surface of greater trochanter	Rotates extended thigh laterally; abducts flexed thigh

Medial thigh muscles: adductors and internal rotators. These powerful muscles help to keep the femur from abducting too much during the swing phase of walking (Figures 8.8 and 8.9). In other words, as you are standing on your left leg and swing your right leg through to step on the right foot, the right adductors help to keep your right leg moving straight ahead instead of wandering off to the right as it swings through, thus creating a more efficient gait. The adductors are strengthened and stretched by standing poses and certain seated poses in which the thighs abduct. Examples include Prasarita Padottanasana, Upavistha Konasana, and Baddha Konasana.

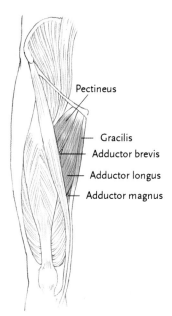

8.8 MEDIAL THIGH MUSCLES

Posterior thigh muscles: hip extensors and knee flexors. Even beginning yoga students become highly aware of their hamstring muscles early in their practice, as they are generally taught to stretch them from the very first class (Figures 8.10 and 8.11). This muscle group is much smaller than the hip flexor–knee extensor group, but it usually receives more attention in yoga class. The hamstrings are strengthened during hip extension against gravity, such as in Urdhva Dhanurasana. They are stretched by hip flexion, especially when the knee is extended. All forward bends stretch the hamstring muscles when the knee is held straight and the hip joint flexed. One example is Paschimottanasana.

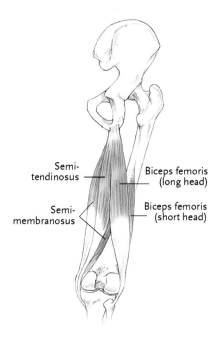

8.10 POSTERIOR THIGH MUSCLES

8.9 MEDIAL THIGH MUSCLES

MUSCLE	ORIGIN	INSERTION	ACTION
Gracilis	Inferior ramus of pubis	Medial aspect of upper tibia below medial condyle	Adducts femur; flexes leg and then medially rotates it
Pectineus	Pectineal line of lateral pubic bone	Between lesser trochanter and linea aspera	Flexes, adducts, and medially rotates femur
Adductor longus	Medial pubis	Lower linea aspera	Flexes, adducts, and medially rotates femur
Adductor brevis	Medial pubis	Middle part of linea aspera	Flexes, adducts, and medially rotates femur
Adductor magnus	Inferior ramus of pubis, inferior ramus of ischium, and tuberosity of ischium	Linea aspera and medial femoral condyle	Adducts femur; upper portion medially rotates and flexes femur; lower portion externally rotates and extends femur

8.11 POSTERIOR THIGH MUSCLES

MUSCLE	ORIGIN	INSERTION	ACTION
Biceps femoris: short head	Linea aspera	By common tendon to lateral side of head of fibula	Flexes leg at knee; after it is flexed, rotates tibia laterally
Biceps femoris: long head	Ischial tuberosity	Lateral side of head of fibula	Extends femur and rotates tibia laterally
Semitendinosus	Ischial tuberosity	Proximal medial tibia	Extends the femur; flexes leg and, after it is flexed, rotates tibia medially
Semimembranosus	Ischial tuberosity	Medial condyle of femur	Extends femur; flexes the leg and, after it is flexed, rotates tibia medially

Pelvic floor muscles. The pelvic diaphragm covers the lower opening at the base of the pelvis to support the abdominal organs and gives support to the pelvic organs (Figures 8.12 and 8.13). The pelvic floor has several openings, including openings for the anus, the urethra, and the vagina. These are the muscles used in Kegel exercises, asvini mudra, and mulabandha. The following muscles contribute to the pelvic floor: levator ani, coccygeus, deep transverse perineus, sphincter urethrae, ischiocavernosus, bulbospongiosus, superficial transverse perineus.

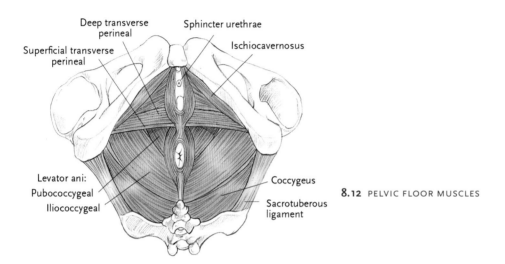

8.12 PELVIC FLOOR MUSCLES

8.13 PELVIC FLOOR MUSCLES

MUSCLE	ORIGIN	INSERTION	ACTION
Levator ani (paired)	Inner superior rami of pubis; inner surface of spine of ischium	Last two coccygeal vertebrae and central tendon of perineum, where pairs meet medially	Supports and slightly raises pelvic floor, resisting increased abdominal pressure downward from above to support abdominal organs; aids in defecation
Pubococcygeus	From line running from pubic symphysis to obturator canal	Central tendinous point of perineum, just anterior to anus	Draws anus toward pubic bone; supports abdominal organs and aids in defecation
Iliococcygeus	Tendon of levator ani and spine of ischium	Last two coccygeal vertebrae	Supports and slightly raises pelvic floor, resisting increased abdominal pressure downward from above

KINESIOLOGY

During the practice of Urdhva Dhanurasana, teachers sometimes notice that their students turn their feet and knees out instead of keeping them straight ahead. This occurs when the students are not using their adductor muscles. Here's what is happening. In order to push up into hip extension into the pose against the downward pull of gravity, the gluteus maximus must be used. The gluteus maximus is a hip extensor and has a secondary action of external rotation as well. When the gluteus maximus contracts, it extends the hip joint and externally rotates it at the same time. In order to counteract this secondary component of the gluteus maximus, the external rotation component must be neutralized by internally rotating.

The adductors are the internal rotators. In order to press the knees toward each other in a straight line, you must activate your adductor muscles. This neutralizes the external rotation component of the gluteus maximus and makes it easier for the pelvis to rotate backward over the femoral heads in the back bend. This is what happens in asana class when a teacher asks you to place a lightweight foam block between your knees in Urdhva Dhanurasana. By pressing on the block, you activate the adductors and thus neutralize the external rotation component of the gluteus maximus.

EXPERIENTIAL ANATOMY

For Practicing

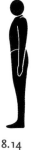

8.14
TADASANA

Applied Practice 1: Experiencing Tight External Rotators in Forward Bends
Prop: 1 nonskid mat
Take Care: If you have any problems with balance, try this near the wall.
ONE OF THE PERSISTENT difficulties yoga students encounter is a limitation of hip flexion because of tightness of the hamstring muscles. Some students find that even with diligent practice the ability to bend forward does not seem to improve very much. Part of the reason could be the tightness of the external rotators.

Here's how it works. While most teachers rightly assume that the action of the external rotators is to externally rotate the femur, these muscles act in another way in daily life. The most common job of the external rotators is to stabilize the pelvis during the swing phase of walking. In other words, when you step out on your right foot, as you transfer your weight onto that foot, there is a period of time in which you are standing on one leg. As your right foot and leg take the weight of your body, the external rotators of the right hip contract to keep the pelvis level to the floor as you swing your left leg through to step on it.

Try it yourself. Stand in Tadasana on your nonskid mat (Figure 8.14). Step on your right foot, and place your fingers over your right rotators, just posterior to the right greater trochanter. As you feel your left leg lift and swing through, you will feel a strong contraction in the right rotators. Therefore every step you take is one in which the external rotators must contract. This strengthens and tightens the rotators, as do poses in which you stand on one leg or strongly externally rotate, as in many standing poses and back bends.

To understand directly how the rotators interfere with hip flexion, try this. Stand in Tadasana and turn your feet out, contracting the external rotators strongly and pressing your buttocks together. Now hold this position of your femurs and try to bend forward into Uttanasana. It will be very difficult, if not impossible. This is simulating the situation of tight external rotators.

8.15
UTTANASANA

Now internally rotate your femurs. This action is the opposite of external rotation and thus will stretch the external rotators. You will find that bending forward is much easier (Figure 8.15). This is because when stretched, the rotators no longer hold the pelvis back, preventing it from rotating over the femoral heads so that hip flexion can occur. Therefore, to improve your forward bends, stretch not only your hamstrings but also your external rotators.

Applied Practice 2: Stretching the External Rotators
Props: 1 nonskid mat
   a bolster (or a blanket folded to 1" x 21" x 28" and rolled firmly from its short end)
Take Care: Skip this practice if it causes pain in your knee joint.

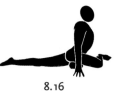

8.16
EXTERNAL
ROTATOR
STRETCH,
WITH BOLSTER

PLACE YOUR BOLSTER crosswise on the mat. Step across the bolster with your right leg, and sit in Eka Pada Rajakapotasana, with your right buttock and upper right thigh resting on the bolster (Figure 8.16).

Your back leg should be straight and internally rotated and your front tibia placed exactly parallel to the short edge of your mat. Pay special attention to this; most students bring the heel in too far instead of making the right tibia parallel to the mat at both the upper and lower tibia.

Make sure that you roll your weight toward the left, lifting your right buttock until it barely presses the bolster, while keeping your right femur firmly on the bolster. This should cause a strong stretch in the right external rotators, especially if you bend forward. Remember to keep breathing as you stretch and to repeat on the other side.

Why this works may be perplexing at first. The rule states that when you want to stretch a muscle, you need to do the opposite of what that muscle does when it contracts. Thus to stretch an external rotator, you need to internally rotate, moving in the opposite direction of the muscle's action. So why are the external rotators stretched in a position of external rotation? This position stretches the external rotators because they are on the posterior surface of the body, and, when you bring the femur into flexion, you begin to stretch the structures on the posterior side.

For Teaching

Applied Teaching 1: Neutral Hip Position in Tadasana

Prop: 1 nonskid mat

Take Care: Make sure that your student's feet are pointing forward and are not turning in or out.

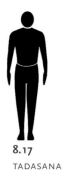

8.17
TADASANA

HAVE YOUR STUDENT stand in Tadasana and first just observe his hip joints from the side and from the front (Figure 8.17). Look at the point where his thighs join his trunk on the anterior side of the body. There should be a small indentation there if the hip joints are in true neutral. Remember, this means that his trochanters are forward of the hip sockets. When he stands with his femurs slightly externally rotated, there will be less or no indentation there.

Now stand behind him, and, after asking permission to touch, place your hands on his greater trochanters. They should be facing slightly anteriorly, due to anteversion of the femoral head in the acetabulum. If they are not, suggest that he slightly internally rotate to bring them into a neutral position.

Applied Teaching 2: Improving Hip Flexion for Supta Padangusthasana

Prop: 1 nonskid mat

Take Care: Do not lie on your back if you are more than four months pregnant.

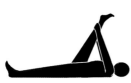

8.18
SUPTA
PADANGUSTHASANA

ASK YOUR STUDENT to lie down on her mat for Supta Padangusthasana (Figure 8.18). First observe as she raises her straight leg up to an angle of 90 degrees. Many students raise the leg with an action that appears as if they are lifting the whole femur at once. Watch this action several times. Now suggest that she lift her femur in a different way: have her imagine that the head of her femur is descending just as she begins the action, in order to allow the rest of the femur to lift. It is as if the femoral head rolls down, back, and out as she raises the thigh and leg up. This way of thinking about the action is more in harmony with what the head of the femur actually does in the movement. Instead, most students just pick up the whole lower extremity and lift it. This way of moving does not allow for the femoral head to move deep into the joint for a mechanically sound movement with increased congruence. This type of movement does not follow the concave–convex law for this joint.

Applied Teaching 3: Improving Forward Bends with Internal Rotation

Prop: 1 nonskid mat

Take Care: Make sure your student is moving from the hip joints to minimize strain to the lower back.

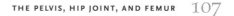

8.19
PASCHIMOTTANASANA

DURING SEATED forward bends, such as Paschimottanasana (Figure 8.19), suggest that the student that internally rotate. One way to do this is to move the inner thigh down firmly toward the floor. When he does this, he will keep the femur in a more neutral position as he bends forward, thus facilitating flexion.

LINKS

Asvini mudra is a seal that is practiced to direct energy in the body. Mudras are practiced to help to channel energy that is moving in one direction in the body to move in another way. *Asvini* refers to the anal sphincter of a horse as it contracts and releases during defecation; *mudra* means "seal." During the practice of yoga poses, Asvini mudra is the contraction of the pelvic floor. This is what women do when they practice Kegel exercises to improve continence and sexual functioning. Asvini mudra also happens spontaneously during the practice of many asana—for example, Urdhva Dhanurasana—due to the strong action of the adductor muscles spilling over to include pelvic floor contraction.

Mula means "root"; Mulabandha is the strong contraction and elevation of the pelvic floor, espe-cially using the pubococcygeus muscle. The difference between Asvini mudra and Mulabandha is twofold. Asvini mudra is a contraction of the pelvic floor to prevent the body's subtle energy from moving down. Mulabandha is the lifting of the pelvic floor, not only to stop energy from moving down but to actively move it upward. The point of Mulabandha is to move the *apana,* or downward feminine energy of the pelvis, upward so it can be maintained in the *kunda*, or vessel of the trunk, and thus will be available for spiritual work.

Mulabandha is usually employed during ad-vanced pranayama techniques, but some systems of yoga deliberately employ it during asana prac-tice. Other systems of hatha yoga believe that this bandha occurs naturally during the practice of asana when alignment of the body is perfected.

The Knee Joint and Leg 9

I THINK THERE IS MORE THAN THE BODY, BUT THE BODY IS ALL
YOU CAN GET YOUR HANDS ON. —IDA ROLF

THE KNEE JOINT is formed by the femur and tibia. Both the fibula and the patella are extra-articular, which means that neither is directly involved in the knee joint proper.

The knee joint is at the apex of the longest lever in the body, the femur, and is a major weight-bearing joint (Figures 9.1 and 9.2). Because of these two facts, the knee is subject to extreme stresses and strains. These stresses occur during both flex-

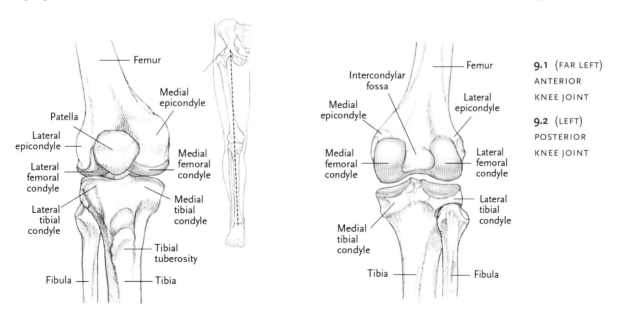

9.1 (FAR LEFT) ANTERIOR KNEE JOINT

9.2 (LEFT) POSTERIOR KNEE JOINT

ion and extension of the knee joint, as well as during the rotational components the joint undergoes. Unfortunately, while the joint is also affected by a number of very powerful muscles, it is not directly supported very much by these muscles. In order to understand the dynamics of this joint, therefore, pay careful attention to its unique structure.

BONES

As we have seen, at the proximal end of the femur, the neck is angled at approximately 130 degrees. Remember that this is the angle between the neck of the femur as is exits the acetabulum and as it bends at the beginning of the shaft of the femur.

If this angle is changed by misplacement of the femoral head in the socket, it can cause alignment difficulties for the knee joint. If this angle is decreased, the head of the femur articulates with the acetablulum in such a way that the femur is in a more abducted position at rest. This condition is referred to as genus varus and is commonly called bow legs. It is more common in men. If this femoral angle is increased, the head of the femur comes into the acetabulum such that the femur is in a more adducted position at rest. This condition is referred to as genus valgus, commonly called knock knees. It is more common in women.

The femur ends in two condyles that are connected to each other on the anterior side but are separate on the posterior side, where they form a hollow called the intercondylar fossa. Just proximal to the condyles are the epicondyles, both lateral and medial prominences that serve as attachment points for soft tissue.

The tibia is the next largest bone in the body after the femur; it forms the other half of the knee joint. Like the distal femur, the superior tibia has two condyles, medial and lateral. The superior surface of these condyles is the surface that is the receiving end of the condyles of the femur. This is the true knee joint. The surface of the medial con-

dyle of the tibia is concave to receive the medial condyle of the femur, while the lateral condyle is less so (Figure 9.3)

On the anterior superior tibia is the tuberosity of the tibia, a large and easily palpable bony prominence that serves as the insertion point for the quadriceps femoris muscle. Find it on yourself now.

Sit comfortably on the floor with your right knee flexed and half way toward your chest, foot resting on the floor. Cup your patella with your right hand so that your fingers are facing in the direction of your foot. Notice the depression at the distal patella. Just below that depression you will feel the bony prominence of the tibial tuberosity sticking out at the center of the tibial shaft.

The lateral surface of the distal tibia is flattened to join with the fibula (Figure 9.4). The distal tibia is elongated to form the medial malleolus, which articulates with the ankle joint.

The fibula joins with the lateral tibia superiorly and forms the lateral part of the ankle joint distally. This part of the fibula is called the lateral malleolus. The fibula is not involved in the knee joint ; its major function is to act as a supporting strut to the lateral leg.

The patella is a sesamoid bone, a type of bone that develops inside a tendon. At the knee joint, this usually happens during the second year of life. The tendon is the quadriceps femoris as it crosses over the joint (Figure 9.5).

The functions of the patella are to cover the knee joint to protect it and to provide increased leverage for the quadriceps femoris muscle as it crosses the knee at the patella. This is how it happens: It is well known that increased leverage is created by the presence of a fulcrum. As the quadriceps femoris tendon passes over the knee joint, it is lifted by the thickness of the patella, which is acting as a fulcrum. This slight elevation of the tendon at the joint creates increased power on knee extension. In fact the patella actually increases the leverage of the quadriceps femoris at the joint from 15 to 40 percent.

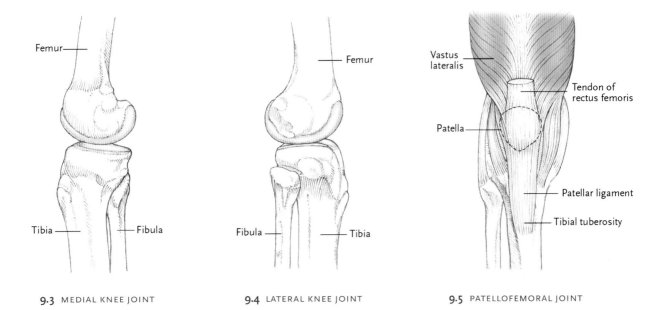

9.3 MEDIAL KNEE JOINT   **9.4** LATERAL KNEE JOINT   **9.5** PATELLOFEMORAL JOINT

When the knee joint is in extension, the patella sits slightly medially. When the knee is in flexion, the patella sits slightly laterally. However, it is not unusual for the patella to drift either too far medially or laterally and remain there. This can sometimes be seen in athletes.

This positional fault of the patella is usually caused by an imbalance in muscular strength in the medial or lateral head of the vasti (the other three heads of the quadriceps femoris) respectively. This condition is called patello-femoral syndrome. Usually it can be improved by specific strengthening exercises for the weak part of the vasti.

JOINTS

The knee joint consists solely of the articulation of the distal femur and the proximal tibia. The center of the joint is to be found on a line drawn directly down from the center of the acetabulum. This line shows that the femur must curve inward from the hip joint to bring the knee joint directly under the acetabulum and that the femur has a medial curve. This is accomplished in part by the medial curve of the femur created by the angle of the neck. This

means that the femoral head sits in the acetabulum at an angle, with the effect that the greater trochanter is actually anterior of the hip joint proper. The knee joint is completed by the presence of the patella, which creates the patellofemoral joint.

The space at the back of the knee is called the popliteal space. Its boundary on the proximal lateral side is the biceps femoris and on the distal lateral side is the lateral head of the gastrocnemius muscle. Its medial borders are the semitendinosus, the semimembranosus, and the medial head of the gastrocnemius. It contains arteries, veins, bursa, the common peroneal nerve, and the posterior tibial nerve.

Another joint around the knee is the articulation of the tibia and fibula. The lateral tibia joins the head of the fibula at a site called the tibiofibular joint. It is a gliding joint with the ability to move slightly anteriorly and posteriorly.

CONNECTIVE TISSUE

The tibia and fibula are joined by the interosseous membrane. It not only keeps the tibia and fibula

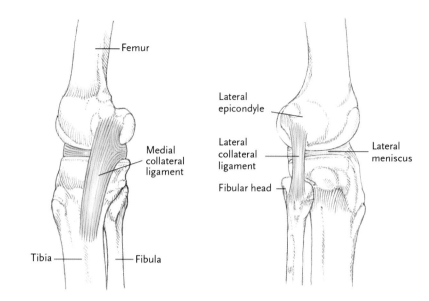

9.6 (RIGHT)
MEDIAL COLLATERAL LIGAMENT

9.7 (FAR RIGHT)
LATERAL COLLATERAL LIGAMENT

connected but also divides the muscles of the leg into anterior and posterior compartments.

The main ligaments of the moving knee joint are called the medial and lateral collateral ligaments (Figures 9.6 and 9.7). These two collateral ligaments give stability to any rotational movements at the joint. The medial collateral ligament is stronger because of the increased need for stabilization on the medial side of the joint, at the site where the femur and tibia join. The distal femur is at an increased angle here, and more movement is allowed than at the lateral knee joint; thus more support is needed. The lateral collateral ligament runs from the lateral epicondyle of the femur to the lateral fibular head and supports the lateral joint.

The medial collateral ligament is the stronger of the two and runs from the medial epicondyle of the femur to the proximal medial shaft of the tibia. Another important distinction between the collateral ligaments at the knee is that the medial collateral ligament is also connected to the medial meniscus. This is one of the factors that allow an increased potential for injury at the medial knee joint, especially twisting injuries during weight bearing.

These types of injuries can occur when the foot is securely planted, the knee flexed, and the femur adducted and internally rotated. In this position, the knee joint is opened at the medial side and made more vulnerable, because during flexion there is less congruence between the femur and tibia and thus less stability. Any added force to the joint at this point, like a tackle in a football game, can cause injury to the medial muscle tendons as well as to the collateral tendon and its adjoining medial meniscus all at once. This injury is called "the unhappy triad of O'Donohue," probably the most colorful name of any orthopedic injury. This connection of muscle tendons, ligament, and meniscus does not exist on the lateral side, which is one of the reasons that the lateral knee is less likely to be injured.

The internal ligaments of the knee joint are called cruciate because they are crossed. They are named for the part of the tibia to which they are connected. Because of the oblique orientation of the cruciates, flexion is allowed and at the same time they restrain tibial-femoral displacement. The anterior cruciate ligament (ACL) is attached to the anterior intercondylar area of the tibia and the lateral meniscus; it runs posteriorly and superiorly to attach to the lateral condyle of the femur (Figure 9.8). The ACL has several functions. It acts as a restraint to hyperextension of the joint. It is

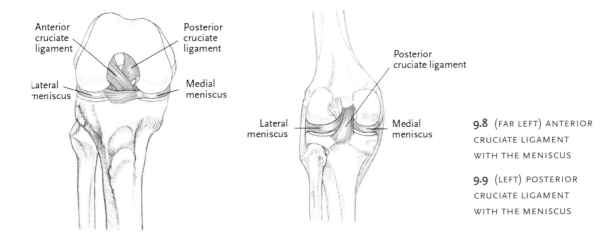

Anterior cruciate ligament

Posterior cruciate ligament

Lateral meniscus

Medial meniscus

Posterior cruciate ligament

Lateral meniscus

Medial meniscus

9.8 (FAR LEFT) ANTERIOR CRUCIATE LIGAMENT WITH THE MENISCUS

9.9 (LEFT) POSTERIOR CRUCIATE LIGAMENT WITH THE MENISCUS

the main structure that restrains anterior tibial displacement, and it limits internal rotation of the tibia. The posterior cruciate ligament (PCL) originates from the posterior intercondylar area of the tibia and attaches at the anterior medial condyle of the femur (Figure 9.9). The PCL passively aids in flexion of the joint

The knee joint has unique connective tissue structures called menisci. These structures act as pads for the knee joint as well as functioning to create a deeper cavity in the superior surface of the tibia for the distal femoral condyles. The menisci maintain an even covering of synovial fluid and thus help keep the joint lubricated for easy movement and reduced friction. Irritation and even destruction of these cartilage surfaces tend to decrease the surface available for weight bearing, thus decreasing this natural lubrication and contributing to degeneration.

Both menisci are thick on their outer rim and thinner in the middle. Each meniscus is attached to a portion of the joint capsule. They move slightly during locomotion. During extension of the knee joint, the mensci move forward slightly, and on flexion they move backward. This is to facilitate the easy movement of the femur on the tibia.

The knee joint has thirteen bursae that act as cushions. They are located anteriorly, laterally, and medially around the joint. The largest of these bur-

sae is located between the patella and the skin. This bursa can be irritated by excessive kneeling, a condition called housemaid's knee. All the bursae function to cushion soft tissue, like tendons and ligaments, from rubbing against bone and increasing the wear on them.

NERVES

The two main nerves around the knee joint are branches of the sciatic nerve. (For more discussion on the sciatic nerve, see chapter 6.) These divisions are called the tibial nerve and the common peroneal nerve. This division occurs just superior to the posterior knee joint.

The tibial nerve is the larger; it passes directly through the popliteal fossa at the back of the joint and continues distally. It is deep in the calf muscles as it descends on the medial side of the Achilles tendon. It finally ends in the connective tissue at the bottom of the foot, where it further divides into the medial and lateral plantar nerves.

The tibial nerve has branches to the knee joint proper and the ankle joint, and it controls the muscles of the calf and muscles of the flexor surface of the foot as well as other muscles in this area.

The common peroneal nerve descends on the lateral side of the popliteal fossa; as it continues it winds around the head of the fibula, courses deep

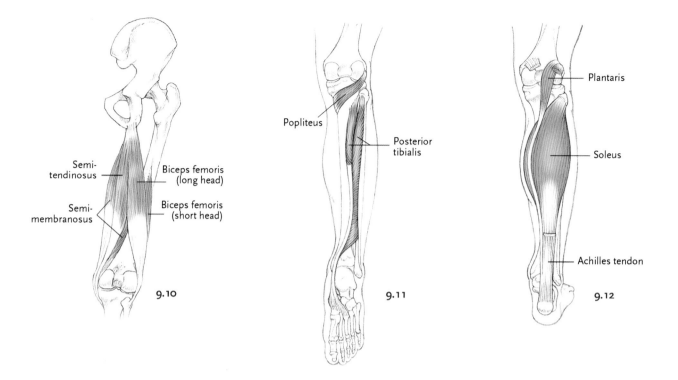

Semi-tendinosus

Biceps femoris (long head)

Semi-membranosus

Biceps femoris (short head)

9.10

Popliteus

Posterior tibialis

9.11

Plantaris

Soleus

Achilles tendon

9.12

9.14   MUSCLES ACTING SPECIFICALLY ON THE KNEE JOINT

MUSCLE	ORIGIN	INSERTION	ACTION
Gastrocnemius, medial head	Posterior medial condyle of femur; medial capsule of knee joint; popliteal surface of femur	Achilles tendon to calcaneus	Flexes knee joint; plantar flexes foot and helps to supinate it; raises heel during walking
Gastrocnemius, lateral head	Lateral condyle of femur, lateral capsule of knee joint	Achilles tendon to calcaneus	Flexes foot and helps to supinate it
Plantaris	Distal lateral supracondylar ridge of femur	Posterior calcaneus	Flexes leg; plantar flexes foot
Popliteus	By strong tendon from lateral condyle and capsule of knee joint	Posterior upper $\frac{1}{3}$ of tibia proximal to popliteal line, superior to soleal line	Weakly flexes leg and rotates it internally

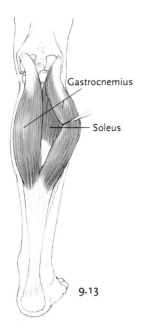

Gastrocnemius

Soleus

9.13

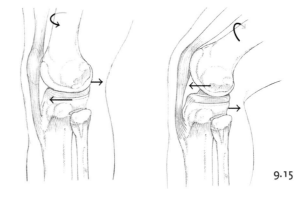

9.15

into the peroneus longus muscle, and divides into deep and superficial branches.

The common peroneal nerve also has branches to the knee joint, as well as to muscles of the lateral and posterior aspects of the leg. Additionally it offers innervation to the tibialis anterior muscles and some of the muscles of the foot.

MUSCLES

The muscles that surround the knee joint are some of the most powerful in the body. The quadriceps femoris, the adductors, and the hamstrings are presented in chapter 8. Here we look at the muscles that are attached to the leg and act upon the knee joint specifically, not the hip joint (Figures 9.10, 9.11, 9.12, and 9.13). The origin, insertions, and actions of these muscles are presented in Figure 9.14.

These muscles are sometimes called secondary knee flexors. When the foot is stabilized or bearing weight, they flex the knee. But when there is no weight on the foot, these muscles will plantar flex the ankle. In other words, they increase the angle between the foot and the leg.

KINESIOLOGY

One of the misconceptions about the knee joint is that it acts as a hinge. Instead, the knee moves with a rolling and gliding action during flexion and extension. During flexion the femur rolls forward on the tibial shelf, while the tibia glides backward on the femur.

The healthily functioning knee joint also has a rotational component that occurs during movement (Figure 9.15). During flexion, there is an unlocking mechanism in which the femur rotates slightly externally on the tibia. This external rotation of the femur on the tibia is the freest at 90 degrees of flexion. This is the position of the front

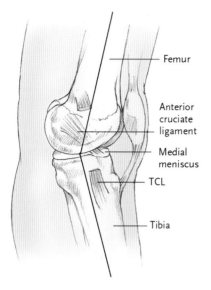

9.16 HYPEREXTENSION OF THE KNEE

Labels on figure: Femur, Anterior cruciate ligament, Medial meniscus, TCL, Tibia

knee joint in Utthita Parsvakonasana or Virabhadrasana I and Virabhadrasana II.

During extension of the knee, the femur rolls backward on the tibial shelf, while the tibia glides forward on the femur. In addition, during extension the femur rotates slightly internally on the tibia in such a way that causes a locking mechanism. This movement is created in part by the shape of the right medial condyle of the tibia and the shape of the medial meniscus. Because of the shape of these structures, the femur moves farther into extension on the medial side of the joint. This contributes to the stability of the joint in extension by helping to create the locking mechanism.

Hyperextension of the knee joint occurs when the backward glide of the tibia on the femur is excessive, so that the joint moves past 180 degrees, or a straight line (Figure 9.16). This hyperextension of the joint contributes to instability in extension and stress on the ligaments of the knee. Hyperextension is inhibited especially by the anterior cruciate ligament but also by the oblique popliteal and collateral ligaments.

Other positional faults of the knee joint are genus valgus and genus varus (discussed on page 110). Genus valgus (knock knees) is more common in women and is caused in part by a decreased angle of the neck of the femur. This causes the knees to come together. A student suffering from genus valgus sometimes is unable to put her feet together in Tadasana because her medial knees meet first. Genus varus (bow legs) is associated with the increased angle of the neck of the femur. It is more common in men. In this case, it might be difficult for the student to put his knees close together in Tadasana.

EXPERIENTIAL ANATOMY

For Practicing

9.17
DANDASANA,
WITH ONE
LEG BENT

Applied Practice 1: Normal Patellar Movement
Prop: 1 nonskid mat
Take Care: Stop immediately if this practice causes any discomfort.
WHEN THE QUADRICEPS muscles are relaxed, the patella is easily moveable. To experience this, sit on your nonskid mat with one leg bent and the other leg extended (Figure 9.17). Relax the quadriceps muscle in the extended leg and grasp the sides of your patella between your thumb and index finger.

Now move your patella gently from side to side; it should move easily and with no pain about an inch in each direction. Now release the patella and contract your quadriceps. You will find that the patella is held firmly against the femur, and you will be unable to move the patella at all. As simple as this technique is, it can be a helpful way to communicate exactly what a contraction of the quadriceps feels like, especially in standing poses.

Applied Practice 2: Testing for Hyperextended Knees
Prop: 1 nonskid mat
Take Care: Do not force your knees to the floor in this test.

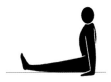

9.18
DANDASANA,
TESTING
FOR KNEE
HYPEREXTENSION

AN EASY WAY to determine if your knees are hyperextended can be done while sitting. Sit in Dandasana on your nonskid mat (Figure 9.18). Make sure your knees are not rotating externally. Now contract your quadriceps very strongly, while keeping your feet completely relaxed. This part is very important; if you dorsiflex your feet, it will interfere with the test.

When you contract your quadriceps, if your heels lift off the floor, it is very likely that your knees have the ability to hyperextend. This can be problematic during the practice of asana, so care should be taken to avoid hyperextending your knees whenever possible.

For Teaching

Applied Teaching 1: Observing the Knee in Tadasana
Prop: 1 nonskid mat
Take Care: Stand on an even surface.

HAVE YOUR STUDENT stand on her mat in Tadasana (Figure 9.19). Make sure that the lateral borders of her feet are parallel to the walls of the room, so that she is not standing in external rotation from her hip.

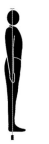

9.19
TADASANA

Now observe her knee joints from the side. If you draw an imaginary vertical plumb line from her outer ear downward through the center of her external shoulder joint and external hip joint, it should pass through the anterior half of her knee joint. Thus in an aligned Tadasana, weight is being carried through the anterior part of the joint.

This relationship means that not only does the structure of the joint itself help to create stability during extension, but that the force of gravity is aiding in creating a position of stability as well. Encourage your student to stand in Tadasana with the knee joint in pure extension, without hyperextending, to provide a position of maximal stability and minimal effort.

Applied Teaching 2: Observing the Knee in Adho Mukha Svanasana
Prop: 1 nonskid mat
Take Care: If your student has wrist pain, practice with the hands on the wall instead.

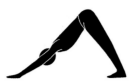

9.20
ADHO MUKHA
SVANASANA

HAVE YOUR STUDENT practice Adho Mukha Svanasana, and, when he is in the pose, stand behind him and observe the backs of his knees (Figure 9.20). Notice two things: first, that the surface at the back of the knee is not parallel to the wall behind you but rather that it is slightly internally rotated. Second, notice that the back of his medial knee is slightly lower than his lateral knee. Both of these phenomena are due to the fact that the femur internally rotates on extension to help to provide stability in the joint. This relationship is the normal shape of the back of the knee in extension.

LINKS

I recommend these two books about knees. Peter Egosue's *Pain Free* (New York: Bantam, 2000) details exercises that I have found very helpful, if not practically miraculous, for students who exhibit a patella that is either internally or externally rotated too much. These exercises help to align the patella, thus increasing the efficiency of the quadriceps muscle at the knee joint and decreasing the strain on surrounding tissues. Sandy Blaine's *Yoga for Healthy Knees* (Berkeley, CA: Rodmell Press, 2005) offers a comprehensive yoga program for pain prevention and rehabilitation.

The Ankle and Foot 10

WE OFTEN IGNORE our feet except when they hurt. We force them into stylish but ill-fitting shoes and walk around on high heels, shifting our weight forward onto the metatarsals, which are not equipped to receive it, and rolling onto the outside of the ankles. We paint our toenails but ignore our flat arches.

On my first trip to India, I was walking in a city garden one day and was struck by the bare wet footprints left by one of the gardeners on the stone pathway. Each footprint looked like the drawing of a perfect foot. Each toe print was round and perfect, the arch was clearly lifted, and the heel print was an even ovoid. After that experience, I began to notice other feet in India and how the wearing of simple sandals had allowed so many people to have wide, strong, and open feet. It was quite a comparison to the Western feet I saw in my yoga class. Those feet had first (big) toes that were often abducted, ankles that were pronated, arches that were fallen. The entire foot was generally misshapen from wearing shoes that confined and restricted.

Luckily, the conscious practice of yoga asana can help us regain healthily shaped feet by stretching and strengthening the muscles of the feet and reminding us to open our toes and stand well. Study this chapter to learn about the structures of the feet and ankles and how to improve your foot function.

BONES OF THE ANKLE

There are fifty-two bones in the feet—about one-fourth of all the bones in the body. The ankle bones, or tarsals, are seven in number. The most superior one is the talus. It is a pivotal bone, connecting the tibia superiorly, the calcaneus distally, and, on the sides, the lateral and medial malleoli. There are no muscles that attach to the talus.

Just distal to the talus is the calcaneus (Figures

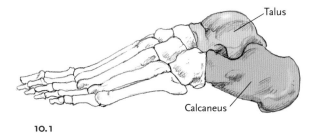

10.1

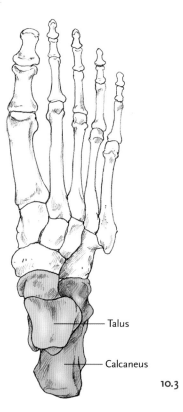

10.3

10.1 and 10.2). This is the largest bone in the foot and therefore is important in weight bearing. The calcaneus is located at the posterior foot and is at the main junction where the weight of the body is translated to the ground (Figure 10.3).

When practicing Tadasana, it is important to understand the weight-bearing function of the calcaneus. Sometimes yoga students are instructed to equalize the weight throughout the foot. But this instruction does not take into account the actual structure of the ankle and foot.

10.1 TALUS AND CALCANEUS, LATERAL VIEW

10.2 TALUS AND CALCANEUS, MEDIAL VIEW

10.3 TALUS AND CALCANEUS, SUPERIOR VIEW

10.4 TARSALS, MEDIAL VIEW

10.5 TARSALS, LATERAL VIEW

10.6 METATARSALS AND PHALANGES, SUPERIOR VIEW

Take a minute to notice your leg, ankle, and foot in standing. The leg joins the ankle at the back of the foot, not at the center in the arch. The large talus and calcaneus are at the back of the foot as well. This is the site of weight transfer, not the middle of the foot. The bones of the posterior foot are the major weight-bearing bones. The smaller bones of the ankle and the long slender bones of the foot (metatarsals) are used mainly for balance and propulsion, though the metatarsal heads do bear some weight. However, if we follow the dictates of structural formation, our weight in standing is meant to be borne mostly at the back of the foot, on the whole heel, which is formed by the calcaneus.

The other function of the calcaneus is to act as a strong lever as the body moves into plantar flexion. This bone is the site of attachment of the Achilles tendon, the largest and strongest tendon in the body. With the strength of the gastroc-soleus muscle focused here, we have tremendous propulsive force for walking and running through the action of the calcaneus. Moving distally, between the talus, the calcaneus, and the metatarsals, in the next layer are the five tarsal bones, which correspond to the instep of the foot (Figures 10.4 and

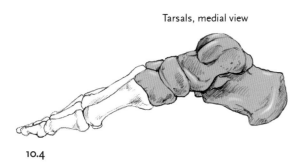

Tarsals, medial view

10.4

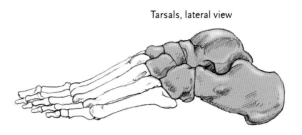

Tarsals, lateral view

10.5

10.5). The navicular is located on the medial side of the foot, between the talus and the cuneiform bones. The navicular articulates with the first, second, and third cuneiforms. The cuboid bone, so named because of its shape, is located on the lateral side of the foot. It articulates with the calcaneus proximally, with the lateral cuneiform and the navicular medially, and with the fourth and fifth metatarsals distally (Figure 10.6).

To find your navicular bone, sit on a chair and cross your right foot over your left leg easily at the knee, so you can see the arch side of your foot. Press your fingers firmly from the medial base of your first toe along the side of the first metatarsal, and then slowly move them proximally toward the ankle. The first prominence you find will be slightly medial; it is the first cuneiform. If you continue to move a short distance in this direction, you will find another prominence about an inch or an inch and a half away; this is the navicular bone.

You can easily locate your cuboid bone as well. Once again sit on a chair and cross your right foot over your left leg easily at the knee. Now run your left fingers firmly along the lateral border of your foot, from your little toe toward your ankle, this time with your left hand. At the proximal end of your fifth metatarsal bone, which forms this border, you will feel a protuberance. You will feel a bit of a "drop off" here at the proximal end of the fifth metatarsal. Move your fingers just proximal to this drop off, and you will find the cuboid bone.

The remaining three tarsal bones are the cuneiform ("wedge-shaped") bones, which create a transverse arch of the foot. The medial cuneiform

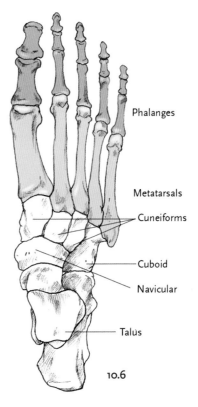

Phalanges

Metatarsals

Cuneiforms

Cuboid

Navicular

Talus

10.6

is the largest and articulates with the navicular, the second cuneiform, and the first and second metatarsals. The intermediate cuneiform is the smallest of the three; it articulates with the navicular, the other two cuneiforms, and the second metatarsal. The last cuneiform is located most laterally of the three cuneiforms, and it articulates with six bones: the navicular, the intermediate cuneiform, the cuboid, and the second, third, and fourth metatarsals. You can palpate the cuneiforms across the top of your medial arch.

BONES OF THE FOOT

There are five metatarsals, numbered from one on the medial side to five on the lateral side. The bodies of the metatarsals are long and slender and slightly curved upward toward the top of the foot; they consist of a proximal base, a body, and a distal head. The first metatarsal is remarkable because it is much thicker and bigger that the other four.

There are fourteen phalanges on each foot. The first toe only has two, a proximal and distal one, while all the other toes have three each. These phalanges as a group consist of three rows: proximal, medial, and distal, according to their location.

JOINTS

The ankle joint is surrounded by a fibrous capsule. It is a hinge joint, consisting of the medial malleolus of the tibia and the lateral malleolus of the fibula, which fits around the talus. The ankle joint dorsiflexes and plantar flexes; it has a large range of movement. In plantar flexion, however the joint is less stable. The movements of the ankle to the foot are supported by a number of ligaments and muscles.

Each foot has thirty-three joints upon which we balance. They are formed into two distinctive longitudinal arches as well as into a series of transverse arches. The first arch is the medial longitudinal arch, the largest and most easily recognizable

one, usually called "the arch of the foot" in asana class. It is formed by the juncture of the calcaneous, the talus, the navicular, the three cuneiforms, and the first three metatarsals. The support of the long arch of the foot is created specifically by the calcaneo-navicular ligament, the long plantar ligament, and the tibialis posterior muscle. The second arch is the lateral longitudinal arch. It is much smaller and extends from the calcaneous to the fifth metatarsal. It can be seen on the outside of the foot.

There are also a series of transverse arches that run from the posterior metatarsal heads to the anterior part of the tarsal bones. In fact, if you put your feet together at the medial longitudinal arch, as is sometimes taught in Tadasana, the transverse arch of the two feet creates a dome. When the body is raised up on one ball of the foot, as in dancing or when wearing high heels, the stress on the arch of the foot is increased many times.

CONNECTIVE TISSUE

Six major ligaments hold the ankle in place. Four are on the lateral side and attach to the fibula, and thus all have "fibula" in their names.

The lateral collateral ligament of the ankle is actually made up of three components—the anterior and posterior talofibular ligaments (ATFL and PTFL) and the calcaneofibular ligament (Figure 10.7). The lateral collateral ligament is the site of 85 percent of ankle sprains. This is true in part

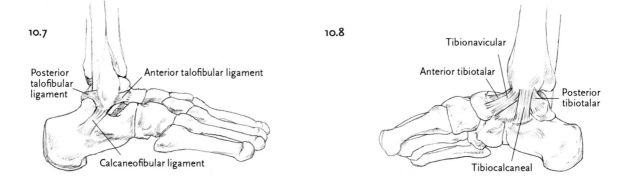

10.7

Posterior talofibular ligament

Anterior talofibular ligament

Calcaneofibular ligament

10.8

Tibionavicular

Anterior tibiotalar

Posterior tibiotalar

Tibiocalcaneal

because the lateral tibia does not extend as far as the medial, thus allowing more instability at the lateral side of the ankle.

The medial collateral ligament of the ankle is also called the tibial collateral ligament, or the deltoid ligament (Figure 10.8). The major function of the deltoid ligament is to prevent too much lateral movement of the talus. It also has an important part to play in plantar flexion.

Remember that the ankle joint is less stable in plantar flexion. This is true because in plantar flexion the narrower part of the talus is held snugly between the medial and lateral malleoli and the arch is stressed. Thus the anterior talofibular ligament is more often the site of injury because it is taut and stressed in plantar flexion. In addition, the inferior talus and the superior calcaneus are held together by the interosseous talocalcaneal ligament as well as the anterior and posterior ligaments between these two bones.

These are the main ligaments of the ankle joint. The other ligaments reinforce the functions already mentioned and can be seen in Figures 10.7 and 10.8. Each foot has over a hundred ligaments, and a detailed explanation of each is beyond the scope of this book. They all function to maintain the stability and integrity of the foot and its arches.

The tarsal and metatarsal joints form gliding joints with many plantar and dorsal ligaments for integrity. Here are the important ones:

► The long plantar ligament runs from the cuboid ridge to the calcaneous and then attaches to the base of metatarsals two through five; it provides medial arch support.

► The short plantar calcaneus cuboid ligament is inferior to the long plantar ligament that runs from the calcaneus to the cuboid.

► The plantar calcanonavicular ligament runs from the calcaneus to the navicular bone to support the head of the talus.

The metatarsophalangeal and interphalangeal joints of the foot are supported by paired collateral ligaments and a deltoid and glenoid ligament as well.

Nerves

The three compartments of the leg are innervated by three different nerves. The anterior compartment muscles are controlled by the tibial nerve, the posterior crural muscles by the deep fibular nerve, and the lateral crural muscles by the superficial fibular nerve (Figures 10.9 and 10.10).

10.7 LATERAL COLLATERAL LIGAMENTS OF THE ANKLE

10.8 DEEP AND SUPERFICIAL LAYERS OF THE MEDIAL COLLATERAL LIGAMENTS OF THE ANKLE

10.9 DEEP NERVES OF THE LEG, ANTERIOR VIEW

10.10 NERVES OF LEG, POSTERIOR VIEW

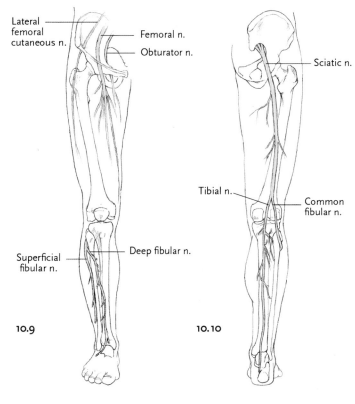

Lateral femoral cutaneous n.

Femoral n.

Obturator n.

Sciatic n.

Superficial fibular n.

Deep fibular n.

Tibial n.

Common fibular n.

10.9

10.10

To observe the route of the nerves around the ankle and foot, please review the Nerves section of chapter 9 and the accompanying diagrams.

It is not uncommon for yoga students and others to feel nerve pain in the plantar surface of the foot (Figure 10.11). One of the most common causes is a neuroma, a thickening of the nerve sheath on the bottom of the foot, which can press on the nerve and cause pain.

Neuromas of the foot are the most common between the metatarsals. One of the reasons neuromas form is from the stress created by poor biomechanics in the foot. When weight is not distributed well through the arch and metatarsals, an irritation to the nerve sheaths may result on the bottom of the foot, causing a neuroma to develop. A frequent solution is surgical excision to remove the neuroma. Unfortunately, however, surgery can create scar tissue in the area and thus exacerbate the condition it was attempting to cure. Learning the correct alignment of the feet in Tadasana and standing poses, as well as practicing strong stretching movements for the plantar surface of the foot, can help prevent this condition and ameliorate it once it has occurred.

MUSCLES

The leg from the knee to the foot is known as the crus, and it is divided into three crural compartments: anterior, posterior, and lateral (Figure 10.12). A complex group of muscles work together in the lower leg to act upon the knee joint, the ankle joint, and the foot. (These do not include the intrinsic muscles of the foot, which are discussed below.)

The anterior compartment contains muscles that dorsiflex the ankle. The posterior compartment contains the plantar flexors of the ankle, the flexors of the toes, and the muscles that invert the foot. The muscles of the lateral compartment evert the ankle.

▶ Anterior crural muscles work as a group to dorsiflex the foot, especially during the swing phase of walking. This is the portion of walking when the back leg is swinging through from the back to the front to become the new stance leg. If the anterior compartment did not dorsiflex the foot at this time, the back foot would hit the floor as it moved forward (Figure 10.13).

▶ Posterior crural muscles, some of the most powerful in the body, are divided into two layers:

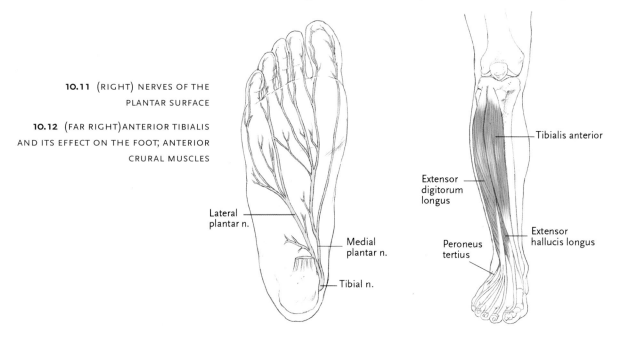

10.11 (RIGHT) NERVES OF THE PLANTAR SURFACE

10.12 (FAR RIGHT) ANTERIOR TIBIALIS AND ITS EFFECT ON THE FOOT; ANTERIOR CRURAL MUSCLES

Lateral plantar n.

Medial plantar n.

Tibial n.

Tibialis anterior

Extensor digitorum longus

Extensor hallucis longus

Peroneus tertius

10.13 ANTERIOR CRURAL MUSCLES

MUSCLE	ORIGIN	INSERTION	ACTION
Tibialis anterior	Lateral condyle and lateral ⅔ of body of tibia	Medial and plantar surface of first cuneiform and base of the first metatarsal	Dorsally flexes and supinates foot
Extensor hallucis longus	Anterior middle ⅓ of fibula and interosseus membrane	Base of distal phalanx of first toe	Dorsally flexes and supinates foot; extends proximal phalanax of first toe
Extensor digitorum longus	Lateral condyle of tibia	Second and third phalanges of four lesser toes	Dorsally flexes and pronates foot; extends proximal phalanges of four lesser toes
Peroneus tertius	Distal anterior fibula	Dorsal fifth metatarsal	Dorsally flexes and pronates foot

superficial and deep. Part of the superficial muscles act upon the knee as well as the foot. The gastrocnemius, plantaris, and popliteus, presented in chapter 9, are discussed again here, with the addition of the soleus. These muscles are sometimes called secondary knee flexors (Figures 10.14, 10.15, and 10.16).

▶ Lateral crural muscles are on the outside of the lower leg. These muscles need to be stretched to practice Padmasana (Figure 10.17).

INTERACTION OF THE ANTERIOR AND LATERAL COMPARTMENT MUSCLES

The anterior tibialis and the peroneus longus and brevis are shaped like a sling under the foot. All these muscles insert on the first metatarsal, and the first two also insert on the first and third cuneiform, respectively. The net effect of this structure is that the anterior tibialis and the peroneals tend to add stability to lateral and medial movements at the ankle. This structure also helps to support the arch. The peroneus longus supports the lateral arch and helps with balance when one is standing on tiptoes (Figure 10.18).

MUSCLES OF THE FOOT

Each foot has nineteen intrinsic muscles. These are muscles that start and stop on the foot itself and do not cross the ankle joint. There is one intrinsic muscle on the dorsal surface of the foot, the extensor digitorum brevis. It arises from the distal and lateral calcaneus and travels across the foot. It has four tendons of insertion; the largest ends at the proximal phalanx of the first toe (sometimes called the extensor hallucis brevis) and the other three tendons insert on the second, third, and fourth toes, on the tendon of the extensor digitorum longus muscle. The action of the extensor digitorum brevis is to weakly extend the proximal phalanges of the first four toes. The tendons of this muscle can often be plainly seen on the top of the foot when the toes are dorsiflexed.

To better understand the muscles on the plantar

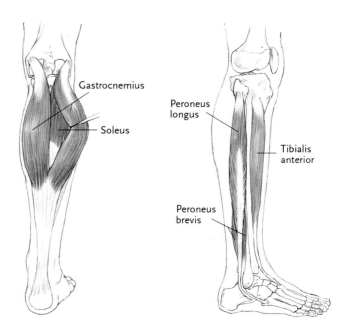

10.14 (RIGHT) GASTROCNEMIUS PULLED BACK TO
SHOW THE SOLEUS AND POSTERIOR COMPONENT

10.18 (FAR RIGHT) PERONEALS AND EFFECT
ON THE FOOT AND LATERAL COMPONENT

10.15 POSTERIOR CRURAL MUSCLES, SUPERFICIAL LAYER

MUSCLE	ORIGIN	INSERTION	ACTION
Gastrocnemius, medial head	Medial condyle of femur; medial capsule of knee joint	Achilles tendon to calcaneus	Flexes knee joint; plantar flexes foot and helps to supinate it
Gastrocnemius, lateral head	Lateral condyle of femur; lateral capsule of knee joint	Achilles tendon to calcaneus	Flexes foot and helps to supinate it
Soleus	Posterior head of fibula; posterior fibula and middle of medial tibia	Gastrocnemius and Achilles tendon to calcaneus	Plantar flexes foot
Plantaris	Distal lateral linea aspera	Posterior calcaneus	Flexes leg; plantar flexes foot
Popliteus	By strong tendon from lateral condyle	Posterior upper third of tibia proximal to popliteal line	Flexes leg and rotates it internally

Muscle	Origin	Insertion	Action
Popliteus	Groove on lateral condyle of femur	Popliteal line on posterior tibia	Flexes leg and rotates it medially
Flexor hallucis longus	Inferior ⅔ of posterior fibula and inferior interosseus membrane	Distal phalanx of first toe with two below	Flexes first toe at interphalangeal and metatarsophalangeal joint
Flexor digitorum longus	Middle posterior tibia inferior to soleal line and fascia covering tibialis posterior	Sole of the foot; divides into four slips	Flexes four lateral toes; helps to propel foot in walking or running
Tibialis posterior	Posterior surface of interosseus membrane; posterior tibia	Tuberosity of navicular bone; plantar surface of cuboid, cuneiforms, and second, third, and fourth metatarsals	Plantar flexes foot at ankle; inverts foot when not bearing weight

10.17 Lateral Crural Muscles

Muscle	Origin	Insertion	Action
Peroneus longus	Head and proximal ⅔ of lateral body of fibula	Lateral base of first metatarsal bone and third cuneiform	Pronates and plantar flexes foot
Peroneus brevis	Distal ⅔ of lateral surface of body of fibula	Tuberosity at base of lateral fifth metatarsal	Pronates and plantar flexes foot

surface of the foot, note that these muscles are arranged into four distinct layers. The bottom of the foot is covered by a thick fascial layer, the plantar fascia, which can sometimes become irritated and create a common condition known as plantar fasciitis.

The four layers work together to flex the toes. The medial plantar muscles control the first toe, the lateral plantar muscles control the little toe, and the intermediate muscles control the medial three toes (Figures 10.19, 10.20, 10.21, 10.22, and 10.23).

KINESIOLOGY

Four movements are allowed at the ankle joint. Plantar flexion, or pointing of the foot, requires

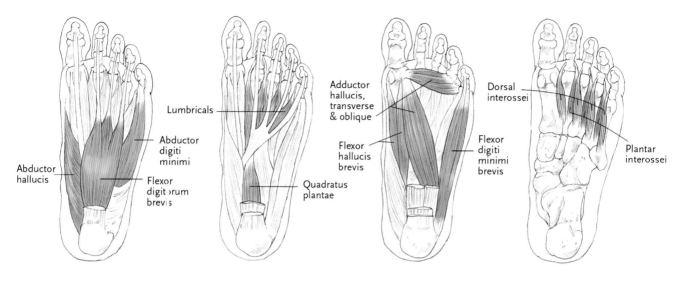

10.19 FOUR LAYERS OF THE BOTTOM OF THE FOOT

10.20 PLANTAR MUSCLES, FIRST LAYER

MUSCLE	ORIGIN	INSERTION	ACTION
Abductor hallucis	Medial calcaneus	Tibial side of base of first toe	Abducts first toe
Flexor digitorum brevis	Medial calcaneus	Sides of second phalanges of four small toes	Flexes second phalanges of four small toes
Abductor digiti minimi	Lateral calcaneus	Fibular side of base of first phalanx of little toe	Abducts fifth toe

some passive joint movement of the talus. In order to plantar flex, the talus must move anteriorly. Because there are no muscles attached to the talus, this movement must be allowed by the laxity in the connective tissue attached to the talus. In a normal ankle joint, there is approximately 45 degrees of plantar flexion.

Dorsiflexion is limited to approximately 20 degrees. To have a full range of dorsiflexion, the talus must glide posteriorly. Dorsiflexion is also limited by tightness in the gastrocnemius and soleus muscles and the Achilles tendon. Many students present with tightness in this area of the body, in part because in our culture we do not often squat. Tightness in this area can also be created by running and other athletic pursuits and by the frequent wearing of high heels. If the knee is bent, the gastrocnemius is stretched, and some increase in dorsiflexion is possible.

A simple stretching exercise can be used to stretch this area, as well as to isolate the stretch of the gastrocnemius and soleus, in order to improve dorsiflexion. Stand facing the wall, with your hands on the wall at shoulder height. Then place

FIGURE 10.21 PLANTAR MUSCLES, SECOND LAYER

MUSCLE	ORIGIN	INSERTION	ACTION
Quadratus plantae	Medial and lateral calcaneus	Tendon of flexor digitorum longus	Flexes distal phalanges of four small toes
Lumbricals	Tendons of flexor digitorum longus	Dorsal surface of first phalanx	Flexes proximal phalanges and extends two distal phalanges of four small toes

FIGURE 10.22 PLANTAR MUSCLES, THIRD LAYER

MUSCLE	ORIGIN	INSERTION	ACTION
Flexor halllucis brevis	Medial cuboid, lateral cuneiform	Medial and lateral sides of base of first phalanx	Flexes proximal phalanx of first toe
Adductor hallucis	Bases of second–fourth metatarsal bones	Lateral side of base of proximal phalanx of first toe	Adducts first toe
Flexor digiti minimi brevis	Base of the fifth metatarsal bone	Lateral side base of the first phalanx of the fifth toe	Flexes proximal phalanx of the fifth toe

FIGURE 10.23 PLANTAR MUSCLES, FOURTH LAYER

MUSCLE	ORIGIN	INSERTION	ACTION
Interosseus dorsales	By two heads from sides of adjacent metatarsals	Bases of first phalanges by two divisions into lateral and medial sides	Abducts toes from longitudinal axis of second toe
Interosseus plantares	Bases and medial sides of bodies of the third to fifth metatarsals	Medial sides of the bases of first phalanges of third to fifth toes	Adducts toes toward axis of second toe

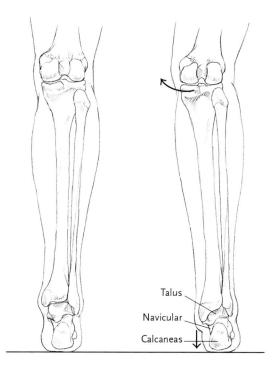

10.24 PRONATION AND ITS EFFECT ON THE POSITION OF THE KNEE

soleus will be felt from the mid-calf area down, the location of the soleus.

The third movement allowed at the ankle joint is supination, which is done by gliding at the subtalar joint, as well as by gliding at the joints between the talus and the calcaneus and navicular bones. This movement is quite free and can be overdone in poses like Padmasana if you go into the pose by pulling on your foot instead of keeping the ankle in neutral and placing the ankle on the opposite thigh. The ability to supinate easily can lead to a sprain of the lateral collateral ligaments of the ankle. Inversion of the foot often accompanies supination of the ankle.

The fourth movement of the ankle is pronation (Figure 10.24). Pronation is allowed by gliding at the subtalar joint, as well as by gliding at the joints between the talus, calcaneus, and navicular bones. Pronation is much less free than supination. Pronation of the ankle can be increased by ligamentous laxity in the foot, creating pronation of the longitudinal arch and thus of the ankle. Pronation of the ankle can directly effect the healthy functioning of the knee joint by causing increased tibial torsion, an increased internal rotation of the tibia on the femur. Eversion of the foot often accompanies pronation of the ankle.

ANKLE SPRAINS

Caution: If you suspect an ankle sprain, send the student immediately for medical attention, including to a therapist who works with connective tissue. A sprained ankle is one of the most under-treated injuries on a long-term basis and can lead to problems with the knee joint.

Ankle sprains are actually tears in the ligamentous support to the joint. They can be partial or, occasionally, complete. Sprains usually occur when the individual steps off an uneven surface or falls during athletic endeavors and lands on the ankle in supination. Pain can be severe, and swelling is

your right foot back about two feet, with your heel turned slightly out. Your front knee should bend directly over the front foot. The stretch is created by making sure your back heel is held firmly on the ground throughout. Hold the stretch for at least 30 seconds. This variation will stretch the gastrocnemius. Remember that the gastrocnemius is a two-joint muscle, and, in order to stretch it, the muscle must be stretched over both the knee joint and the ankle joint.

To stretch the soleus, a one-joint muscle, assume the same position facing the wall. This time, however, bend your back knee as well as your front knee. Be very careful to keep your back heel on the floor when you bend this knee, however. Bending the back knee will release the stretch of the gastrocnemius over the knee joint, thus emphasizing the stretch of the soleus muscle over the ankle. The first stretch of the gastrocnemius will be felt throughout the calf area. The second stretch of the usually immediate, although the amount of pain may not be correlated to the degree of injury.

One way to know if your student has a mild ankle sprain is to ask her to perform the following. Have her sit in a chair and lift the affected side off the floor. Now have her move her ankle passively with her hand to see if that elicits pain. Pain on active movement could be caused by a sore or injured muscle and not a sprain. She or another trained person can now move her foot gently so it plantar flexes and supinates at the same time. If this creates pain, it is likely that there is an injury to the ATFL, and she should seek medical attention.

EXPERIENTIAL ANATOMY

For Practicing

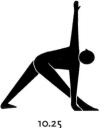

10.25
UTTHITA
TRIKONASANA

Applied Practice 1: Foot Position in Standing Poses

Prop: 1 nonskid mat

Take Care: When you turn the front foot out, also drop the femur toward the back of your thigh. Make sure that this movement does not create pain in the inner knee structures.

ONE OF THE MOST important focus points in standing poses is the position of the feet. In Utthita Trikonasana, for example, the front thigh is rotated externally about 90 degrees, so the foot is facing out to the side and the back foot is rotated medially and facing inward about 45 degrees (Figure 10.25). On the one hand, many students find it easy to supinate the front foot and pronate the back foot. On the other hand, students who are limited in internal rotation because of tight hip external rotators sometimes pronate the front foot. This tightness in the back hip can result in a supinated back foot, as the student tries in vain to externally rotate the tight back hip and ends up instead supinating the ankle and foot.

During your practice of Utthita Trikonasana, observe your front foot after you have turned it out from the hip. Place weight both on the ball of the first toe at the proximal end of the first phalanx and equally on the lateral border of the calcaneus.

Now observe your back foot. If you feel steady, close your eyes and feel where the weight is on the foot. You may need to press a little more weight on the outside of your back foot to keep the relationship of even pressure on the first metatarsal bone and the center of the calcaneus. This will help to create a diagonal relationship of pressure across the foot that will keep your ankle in a neutral position, neither supinated nor pronated.

10.26
DANDASANA

Applied Practice 2: Foot Position in Seated Forward Bends

Prop: 1 nonskid mat

Take Care: Avoid this practice if you have disc disease in your lower back.

SIT ON YOUR nonskid mat in Dandasana (Figure 10.26). Place your first metatarsals together and your heels slightly apart. Now notice the angle of the first metatarsals. While keeping them together, slightly evert the feet, that is, press the first metatarsals away from you and draw the fifth metatarsals toward you. This should make the bottom of the feet a bit uneven.

However, when you slightly evert the feet in Dandasana, notice how that action affects your whole lower extremity, causing it to roll slightly internally, the knees to straighten, and the inner calf to press the floor. This position is neutral for the lower extremity in forward bends. Maintain this position of the feet as you bend forward with an exhalation into Paschimottanasana (Figure 10.27). Remember to keep pressing your first metatarsal bones forward as you descend into a forward bend; imagine that they are leading you into the pose. Remember this position of the feet in all seated forward bends.

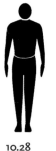

10.27
PASCHI-
MOTTANASANA

For Teaching

Applied Teaching: Foot Position in Tadasana

Prop: 1 nonskid mat

Take Care: Stand on an even surface.

HAVE YOUR STUDENT STAND in Tadasana on a nonskid mat (Figure 10.28). Suggest that he place his feet about 6 to 8 inches apart for the purpose of this lesson. First observe the lines along his fifth metatarsals. Make sure that he has placed the lateral borders of his feet parallel to the edges of his mat. He will likely need to move his heels externally to create this line. Most students stand with their heels too close together and thus in a position of external rotation of the thigh, leg, and foot.

Notice the general appearance of his foot, the shape of the arches, and if the toes are straight out or if the first toe is abducted and the other toes adducted. Now move behind him and observe the Achilles tendons. In an aligned foot, the Achilles tendons are vertical. You may want to suggest that he move the feet in what ever way is necessary to create a vertical line with the Achilles.

Now observe his medial and lateral malleoli. Are they parallel to the floor? If not, have him shift his weight or modify his foot position to make this happen. Finally, after asking permission to touch, you may want to stand behind him and press down firmly on the tops of his shoulders to see if he can easily bear your weight. If the student has aligned feet, he will bear this weight with no effort.

10.28
TADASANA

LINKS

Young children often appear to have flat feet because they have extra fat in their arches. As they mature, the natural arch usually appears. However, if you are concerned that a two- or three-year-old does indeed have flat feet, have the child examined by a health care professional.

With yoga games, the 5-minute class, relaxation games, and more, *Create a Yoga Practice for Kids,* by Yael Calhoun, M.Ed., M.S., and Matthew R. Calhoun (Santa Fe, NM: Sunstone Press, 2006), makes yoga fun for children and their parents and teachers.

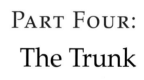

PART FOUR:
The Trunk

The Abdomen 11

TRUST YOUR BELLY.

—JUDITH HANSON LASATER

DURING MY FIRST months of studying asana, I took a kundalini yoga class. I was introduced to my "core" at that class by the practice of powerful breathing techniques that were focused on impacting the *kunda,* or vessel, which anatomists call the thorax and abdomen. We were taught in that class the importance of the energy of the kunda. Since that time, I have paid increasing attention to my organs and how they are affected by asana practice.

We begin our discussion of the trunk with a brief introduction to the anatomy of the chest and belly. While these areas do not generally initiate movement, as do the vertebral column or arms and legs, the core, or belly, receives the powerful effects of all asana. If the organs in the center of our body are healthy, then we are likely to be healthy as well.

The abdomen is a complex area anatomically, and it has emotional aspects as well. We use expressions like "I knew in my gut it was a good idea," or "My stomach is in a knot." Research has shown that these expressions actually express physiological truths. Apparently there are receptor sites in the abdomen that respond to the same neurotransmitters as the brain does. So it turns out that when we say we had a gut sense about something, we did. Perhaps this sense of knowing can be defined as intuition. Whatever we call it, paying attention to our body's sensations both in practicing and in teaching yoga is an important skill to cultivate and honor.

The size and shape of the abdomen receives a lot of attention in our fitness-conscious society, and a common belief about the abdominal muscles is that they should be rock hard. We often judge people negatively who have a rounded or soft belly. However, there is a difference between an abdomen with toned muscles and yet a natural rounded shape and one that is contracted and tightly pulled in. Holding the abdominal muscles in a hard and contracted manner can interfere with breathing and digestion, among other functions.

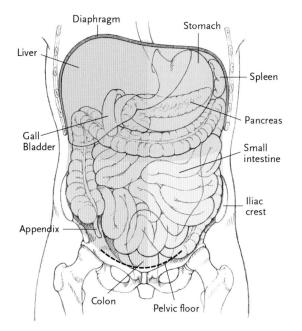

11.1 ABDOMINAL ORGANS, ANTERIOR VIEW

of the organs to press the fluids out. These classical techniques and their effects on the abdominal organs have not yet been proven in scientific studies. Nonetheless, it is useful for yoga teachers to understand these classical benefits and then teach the appropriate asana that affect the health of the organs in general.

To begin to understand the anatomy of the abdomen, remember that the abdomen cavity proper is divided into four quadrants: upper right and left, and lower right and left (Figure 11.1). For example, the appendix is located in the lower right quadrant, and the stomach is in the upper left quadrant. Take some time now to familiarize yourself with the location of these and the other abdominal organs and to commit these locations to memory. This understanding will help you to visualize the location of the abdominal organs during your own practice and when teaching others.

BONES

The abdomen is the largest single cavity in the body. It is bounded on the anterior surface by the sternum and pelvis, specifically the pubic area, on the lateral sides of the body by the ilia, and on the posterior side by the lumbar vertebrae and the sacrum. The superior boundary of the abdomen is the diaphragm muscle, while the inferior boundary is the pelvic floor. Within this area lie all the organs of digestion, assimilation, elimination of solid and liquid waste, procreation, and one site for the production of red blood cells (the spleen).

JOINTS

The abdominal cavity has no joints, per se, but the movements created by the contraction and relaxation of the abdominal muscles affect the joints of the thoracic, lumbar, and sacral spine as well as the costal joints. See chapters 5, 6, and 7 to review these movements.

Try this experiment. Stand in Tadasana on your nonskid mat and contract your abdomen. Now try to take a deep breath. Release the abdomen and try again. The difference is profound. A naturally toned abdomen is not tense. It simultaneously provides support for the abdominal organs and spine and holds the organs in place, while allowing free and easy breathing.

In traditional yoga teachings, the abdomen is also the location of several of the *chakras*, the subtle energy centers. In fact, when asana practice focuses on the chakras, the goal is release, awareness, and organ health, not just muscular strength of the belly.

Because classical yoga asana teachings focus on the abdominal organs as a key to health, the poses are designed to affect them through a "squeezing and soaking" technique. This means that some poses alternatively increase the blood flow to the abdominal organs, thus "soaking" them with nutrients, and other poses create a "squeezing"

CONNECTIVE TISSUE

The abdominal cavity is lined with a serous membrane called the peritoneum. This membrane, like other serous membranes in the body, is strong and elastic and secretes moisture. This wetness eases the slight movements of the organs inside the abdominal cavity. Besides performing the function of lining the abdominal cavity, the peritoneum has folds that are attached both to the posterior wall of the abdomen and to the organs to help hold them in place. These folds are called the mesentery. The largest fold of the mesentery is called the greater omentum, which attaches in several layers to the stomach, the intestines, and the transverse colon. The lesser omentum connects the liver, stomach, and part of the transverse colon. Both are highly vascularized.

Another connective tissue of note is the linea alba, literally, "white line" (Figure 11.2). The linea alba is a flat band of connective tissue where the rectus abdominus, the internal and external oblique muscles, and the transverse abdominus join into a single tendinous band. This band attaches superiorly from the xiphoid process and inferiorly to the symphysis pubis.

The stress placed on the abdominal wall by the growing fetus during pregnancy stresses the linea alba as well. In fact, it is not uncommon for the two sides of the abdominal muscles to separate slightly at the linea alba. In order to prevent this from happening, make sure that your yoga students do not overstretch their abdominal muscles during pregnancy. This would mean no back bending poses after the first trimester of pregnancy, as well as no poses that cause a pulling on the abdominal muscles at either the xiphoid process or the pubic symphysis.

The inguinal ligament is a significant ligament of the abdominal area. It is created by the lower border of the connective tissue of the external oblique muscle. It is attached to the anterior superior iliac

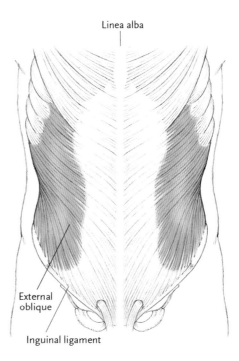

11.2 ABDOMINAL MUSCLES, SUPERFICIAL VIEW

spine and the pubic tubercle. Under this ligament pass nerves, arteries, veins, and lymphatic vessels from the lower extremity to the abdominal cavity. The inguinal area is also the occasional site of herniation, when a portion of abdominal contents can bulge out under the ligament. This usually requires surgical repair.

Yoga students can compress the inguinal area by practicing deep flexion of the hips, as in squatting poses. Take care not to hold these poses for too long. One of the symptoms of this compression is a surface numbness around the anterior superior thigh. This usually resolves quickly when the pose is released. If this surface numbness does not vanish, check with your health care professional.

NERVES

While the abdomen is replete with nerves, by far the most important nerve in the area is the vagus nerve (Figure 11.3). The word *vagus* is related to the word *vagabond,* which means "to wander." The

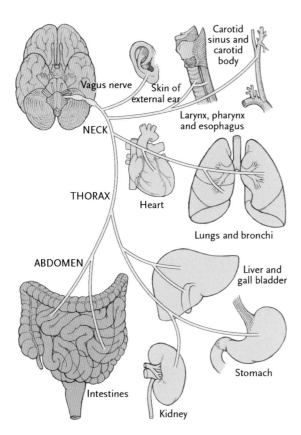

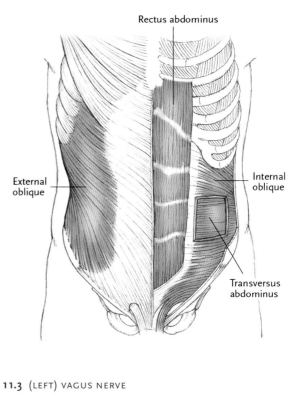

11.3 (LEFT) VAGUS NERVE

11.4 (ABOVE) ABDOMINAL MUSCLES: INTERNAL
OBLIQUES AND TRANSVERSUS ABDOMINUS

vagus nerve has the greatest distribution of all the twelve cranial nerves.

The vagus nerve is the tenth cranial nerve. It arises from the base of the brain and courses distally and inferiorly to help to control virtually all the thoracic and abdominal organs. It controls most parasympathetic functions as it passes through the neck, thorax, and abdomen. Additionally, the vagus nerve influences the skin of the external ear and the mucus membranes of the pharynx, larynx, bronchi, lungs, heart, esophagus, stomach, intestines, and kidney. It also affects the heart muscle and the smooth muscles of the entire digestive tract.

The vagus nerve itself makes up most of the parasympathetic nervous system (PSNS). The PSNS is activated by muscle relaxation, a reclining or head-down position, and by exhalation, among other stimulants. This is part of the reason we experience asana practice as calming; during practice we are stimulating the parasympathetic nervous system by stretching, inversions, and exhaling.

MUSCLES

The abdominal muscles create a basket-weave effect on the anterior abdomen. The rectus abdominus is a vertical muscle and is on the most superficial layer. The external oblique muscles run from the lateral side to the medial at an angle; the next layer is the internal oblique muscles, which run from the inside toward the outside. The last layer is the transversus abdominus, which crosses the abdomen horizontally. These muscles can be studied in Figures 11.4 and 11.5.

MUSCLE	ORIGIN	INSERTION	ACTION
Rectus abdominus	By tendons from crest of pubis and symphysis pubis	Cartilages of fifth, sixth, and seventh ribs; xiphoid process	Flexes vertebral column; stabilizes trunk; compresses abdominal contents; can help in forced exhalation
External oblique abdominus	Inferior border of lower eight ribs	Outer lip of iliac crest; anterior and superior iliac spine and aponeurosis, which inserts into linea alba	Compresses abdominal contents; can help in forced exhalation; one side contracting singularly side bends and rotates vertebral column, bringing same side shoulder down; with both muscles contracting, flexes vertebral column
Internal oblique abdominus	Lateral inguinal ligament; lateral iliac crest; thoraco-lumbar fascia	Last three or four ribs; linea alba; pubic crest; pectineal line	Compresses abdominal contents; can help in forced exhalation; one side contracting singularly side bends and rotates vertebral column, bringing opposite shoulder down; with both muscles contracting, flexes vertebral column
Transverse abdominus	Lateral inguinal ligament; anterior iliac crest; thoraco-lumbar fascia; cartilages of last six ribs	Linea alba; abdominal aponeurosis; pubis	Compresses abdominal contents; can help in forced exhalation
Pyramidalis	Anterior pubis	Linea alba, midway between navel and pubis	Tenses linea alba

KINESIOLOGY

The function of the woven structure of the abdominal muscles is threefold. The abdominal muscles are necessary to help support the upright vertebral column. They hold the abdominal organs in place. And they are major stabilizers for most of the actions of the body.

It would be good at this point for you to review the concept of stabilization presented in chapter 2. Stabilization is the major function of the abdominal muscles. They work together to approximate, or bring together, the rib cage and pelvis to offer stability to the trunk and vertebral column during the movements of asana and in daily life.

To experience the abdominal muscles as stabilizers, lie down on a comfortable surface. After taking a breath or two, place one hand over your navel area. Now lift your head off the floor, and notice the contraction of the abdominal muscles under your hand. This is not because the abdominals are acting as prime movers to lift the head. They are not connected to the neck, so cannot affect the cervical spine. Rather the abdominals contract in this movement to hold the ribcage still, so that the neck flexors can be more effective in flexing the neck. Because the abdominals are mainly used as stabilizers, challenging them as stabilizers is the most effective way to strengthen them.

To stretch the abdominals, the student must perform a back bend. This moves most of the origins and insertions of the abdominal muscles apart—the definition of stretching. However, some yoga teachers suggest that their students actually flex the lumbar spine ("tuck the tailbone") during back bends such as Ustrasana and Urdhva Dhanurasana. Not only does flexing the lumbar spine during a back bend interfere with the lumbo-sacral rhythm (see chapter 7), it also does not allow the abdominals to be fully stretched.

The abdominal muscles frequently interact with the psoas group (psoas major, psoas minor, and iliacus) to promote flexion of the trunk, especially when attempted in a supine position. To experience how this works, sit on a nonskid yoga mat or comfortable carpet, with your legs straight out in front of you. Place your arms in flexion at shoulder height. Now, breathing easily, roll down slowly toward the floor. Note the action of your abdominal muscles as they undergo a lengthening contraction. Once on the floor, bend one knee and roll to the side to return to the sitting position.

Now place the soles of your feet together in a relaxed Baddha Konasana position, and begin to roll down. Remember to breathe and to keep your knees down as much as you can. You will no doubt find this attempt much more difficult. This is because, by changing your leg position, you have put your psoas group at a mechanical disadvantage, and it cannot lend its strength to the descent. In this new attempt, the abdominals are obliged to do all the work of controlling the descent against gravity.

It is important to fully engage the abdominals when using the psoas group to control this movement in order to keep the lumbar spine in flexion. If the abdominals are not working well here, then it is possible for the student to rely on the psoas group too much. When this happens, the lumbar spine could be in too much extension and could suffer strain while the student is rolling down.

EXPERIENTIAL ANATOMY

For Practicing

11.6
NAVASANA

Applied Practice 1: Navasana
Prop: 1 nonskid mat
Take Care: Avoid this pose during the second and third trimesters of pregnancy and if lower back pain is present.

SIT ON a nonskid mat that you have folded in half. Bend your knees to your chest and rock backward, balancing on your tailbone. Now hold the back of the right knee with your right hand and the back of your left knee with your left hand (Figure 11.6). Keep your lumbar spine in flexion, and slowly straighten one knee and then the other. Place your arms at your side, in flexion and parallel to the floor, and balance. It is important to the health of your lumbar spine, and in order to maintain the integrity of the pose, that you remain in flexion, using the strength of your abdominals and hip flexors. Do not lift your chest; this extends the lumbar spine and puts the abdominals at a mechanical disadvantage. When this happens, the abdominals are not able to hold the position very well, and stress is added to the extensors of the lumbar spine and the other structures of the lower back.

Applied Practice 2: Twisting from the Belly in Marichyasana III
Prop: 1 nonskid mat
Take Care: Avoid this twist if you have sacroiliac dysfunction, diagnosed disc disease, or are pregnant.

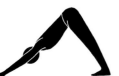

11.7
MARICHY-
ASANA III

MOST OF US practice seated twists by thinking of twisting from the vertebral column. Kinesiologically speaking, the vertebral column twists mainly in the cervical and thoracic regions and minimally in the lumbar spine. (The importance of keeping the pelvis and the sacrum together in twisting is discussed in chapter 7.) To facilitate the maximum twisting from the column that will simultaneously protect the sacroiliac joint, imagine that your twist comes from the abdomen.

Sit in Dandasana on your nonskid mat. On an exhalation, bend your right knee and hold your right leg with your left arm, while you lean back on your right arm for support. As you begin to twist, exhale strongly and then twist with your breath exhaled (Figure 11.7). Imagine that all the twisting is coming from your abdomen; invite your abdominal organs to twist into the spiral of the pose. Exhale another time and, once again, after the exhalation, imagine you are moving your belly organs into the twist. Let the organs lead the twist, and let the vertebral column follow. Notice the feeling of completeness that this way of twisting generates. Be sure to repeat to the other side.

For Teaching

Applied Teaching 1: Abdominal Muscles in Adho Mukha Svanasana
Prop: 1 nonskid mat
Take Care: Avoid this pose after the first trimester of pregnancy or if there are any concerns about inverting the head or body.

11.8
ADHO MUKHA
SVANASANA

HAVE YOUR STUDENT start from her hands and knees on her nonskid mat in preparation for Adho Mukha Svanasana. Now she should exhale and invite her abdominal organs to move upward toward her spine. Her abdominals are definitely contacting here, but she should think that the action is coming from the organs instead. This will change the quality of the movement and increase internal awareness.

As she exhales, ask her to continue lifting, so that her arms straighten but the weight stays forward on her hands and arms. Ask her to inhale and consciously release her abdominal muscles and thus allow her belly organs to drop and the lumbar spine to come into a slight back bend. As she exhales, suggest that she press her heels toward the floor and move backward, to place most of the weight on her legs. This way of coming into

Adho Mukha Svanasana will help your students feel more aware of the action of their abdominal muscles as stabilizers in asana practice.

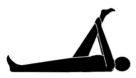

11.9 SUPTA
PADANGUSTHASANA

Applied Teaching 2: Abdominal Muscles in a Straight Leg Raise (SLR)
Props: 1 nonskid mat • 1 blanket
Take Care: Avoid SLRs if you have acute lower back pain.

WHEN YOU ARE teaching your students to raise one leg from a supine position (as in Supta Padangusthasana, Figure 11.9), it is important that they engage their abdominal muscles as well as the psoas group to bring the lumbar spine into flexion, thus stabilizing the pelvis. This will create an action that is done purely at the hip joint, without added stress to the lumbar spine caused by the weight of the leg as it is lifted upward.

As your student prepares to raise one leg from the supine position, be sure he exhales, pulls inward and downward on his abdominal muscles, rocks the pelvis backward, moves the posterior superior iliac spine (PSIS) down toward the floor, and thus feels the top of his sacrum on the floor. Keeping this part of the body down will not only help to strengthen the abdominal muscles in their role of stabilizers but also will protect the lower back. Remember that the abdominals cannot work well as stabilizers unless they are contracting, and this action is best accomplished with a slightly concave abdomen. However, at no time should this contraction interfere with breathing.

LINK

For a new perspective on the belly, see Lisa Sarasohn's *Woman's Belly Book: Finding Your Treasure Within* (Novato, CA: New World Library, 2006). The images, both visual and verbal, are unique and thoughtful.

The Diaphragm 12

THERE IS NO QUESTION THAT THE THINGS WE THINK HAVE A TREMENDOUS
EFFECT UPON OUR BODIES. —C. EVERETT KOOP, M.D.

YEARS AGO I was teaching Tadasana and suggested that the students in the class imagine a relaxed diaphragm muscle, one that felt "dropped down." Suddenly a woman ran from class. After class she told me that when she relaxed her diaphragm, she felt the need to vomit. I was surprised at the ferocity of her reaction but not at the reaction itself. Many of us hold tension in the chest and belly. We restrict our breathing and thus our ability to take in life and give it back out. Breathing is the first act we perform at birth, and at death, the final stopping of breath signals our end. Breathing is even more important for the yoga student; the diaphragm muscle is primary in the practice of pranayama. It is integral to and effected by the practice of asana as well, and it is often a part of the beginning of a meditation session, or the very object of meditation itself. For these reasons, understanding the functioning of the diaphragm is critical for yoga teachers and practitioners.

The diaphragm is significant in the body because it divides the largest two cavities: the thoracic and the abdominal. It is the major muscle that drives respiration. It contracts and relaxes rhythmically nonstop twenty-four hours a day, just like the heart muscle, and it never fatigues.

BONES

The diaphragm is attached to the xiphoid process of the sternum and the inner surfaces of the costal cartilages of the lower six ribs (Figure 12.1). The bodies of the first three lumbar vertebrae are also attached to the diaphragm. It becomes obvious, therefore, that asana involving the placement of these bones can facilitate or inhibit the function of the diaphragm.

JOINTS

The facet joints of the thoracic and lumbar spines, as well as the costovertebral joints, all play a part

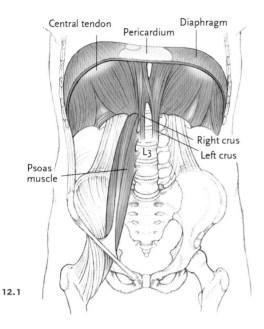

12.1

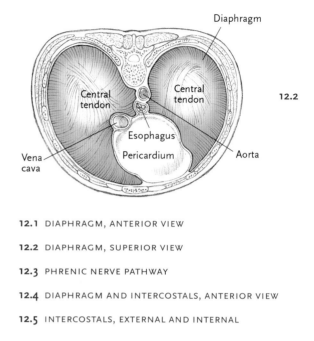

12.2

12.1 DIAPHRAGM, ANTERIOR VIEW

12.2 DIAPHRAGM, SUPERIOR VIEW

12.3 PHRENIC NERVE PATHWAY

12.4 DIAPHRAGM AND INTERCOSTALS, ANTERIOR VIEW

12.5 INTERCOSTALS, EXTERNAL AND INTERNAL

in the mobility of the diaphragm and therefore in the depth and quality of breathing. In order to improve your ability to breathe deeply, these joints must be mobile. Back bending asana, either active or supported, tend to open these joints. Even the practice of Tadasana can help improve breathing by positioning the diaphragm in a neutral position. These joints tend to lose flexibility with age, thus interfering with the excursion of the diaphragm.

CONNECTIVE TISSUE

At the posterior diaphragm are two tendinous structures called crura. The right crus arises from the intervertebral discs and vertebral bodies of the first three lumbar vertebrae. The left crus arises from the intervertebral discs and vertebral bodies of only the first two lumbar vertebrae. Both insert into the clover-shaped central tendon of the diaphragm.

This central tendon of the diaphragm is where the muscle inserts upon itself (Figure 12.2.) The central tendon is an aponeurosis that is located just distal to the pericardium, the covering of the heart; the fascial tissue of the thorax connects the diaphragm to the pericardium. The fascia of the abdomen also connects the vertebrae, the psoas muscles, and the kidneys to the diaphragm at the muscular insertions. In fact, basically all organs both above and below the diaphragm area are connected to the diaphragm in some way, and thus the act of respiration moves them all.

The diaphragm has several openings to allow for the passage of important structures (Figure 12.2). The biggest three are the opening for the aorta, as it descends from the heart through the thorax to abdomen, where it splits into other structures; the opening for the esophagus; and the opening for the vena cava, which is the vein bringing blood from the lower body to the heart. There are also openings for the passage of nerves and smaller veins.

NERVES

The major motor nerve to the diaphragm is the phrenic nerve (Figure 12.3). *Phrenic* is related to the word *frantic*. In Greek, *phren* has as its secondary meaning "the mind, as the seat of the intellect or the heart as the seat of the passions."

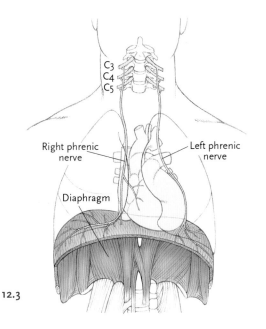

12.3

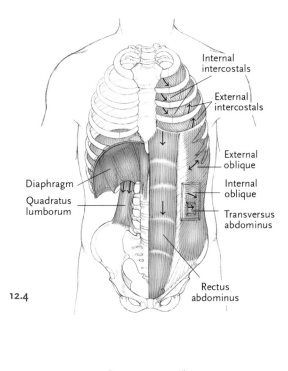

12.4

The phrenic nerve arises from fibers of the third, fourth, and fifth cervical nerves on both sides of the neck. Therefore there are two phrenic nerves, the right and the left. The left phrenic nerve is actually longer, in part due to the placement of the heart.

MUSCLES

Besides the diaphragm itself, other muscles are involved in respiration. These are the external and internal intercostals and the abdominal muscles (Figure 12.4).

The external intercostals run from rib to rib. They originate from the distal rib of the pair and are attached to the superior rib above it. When the external intercostals contract, they draw the ribs together (Figure 12.5). The internal intercostals arise from the inner surface of the ribs and corresponding costal cartilage and insert into the cranial border of the rib below. When the intercostals contract, they draw the ribs together. But the result of this action is slightly more complicated and is discussed in the Kinesiology of Breathing section in this chapter.

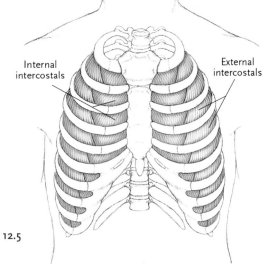

12.5

Three other important muscles that aid in respiration are the serratus posterior superior, the serratus posterior inferior, and the quadratus lumborum. The first arises from the ligamentum nuchae, the spinous processes of C7 through T2, and the supraspinal ligament. It inserts into the superior borders of the second through the fifth ribs. When it contracts, the serratus posterior superior raises the ribs to which it is attached.

The serratus posterior inferior originates from the last two thoracic and first two lumbar vertebrae and from the supraspinal ligament. It inserts into the inferior borders of the last four ribs. When it contracts, this muscle counteracts the inward pull of the diaphragm by pulling the ribs outward and downward. The third muscle, the quadratus lumborum, is discussed in chapter 8.

KINESIOLOGY OF BREATHING

When the diaphragm is stimulated to contract by the phrenic nerve, it descends and moves down from its resting dome shape to a flatter one, increasing its circumference as it does so. This contraction creates an enlargement of the pulmonary space, thus causing the air to enter the lungs due to the drop in pressure inside the lungs compared with the outside pressure. This expansion of the lungs is helped also by the adherence of the covering of the lungs to the lining of the thorax. This adherence causes the lungs to be pulled up and out into expansion with the expansion of the bony thorax.

Exhalation begins when the diaphragm ceases contracting and begins to return to its resting position. It is aided in this by the contraction of the internal intercostals and by the elastic recoil of the lungs and ribs. The quadratus lumborum fixes the last rib and holds it down, so when the internal intercostals contract they bring the ribs down toward it, thus helping the body to exhale the breath.

These actions of the intercostals and other accessory muscles of respiration are greatly increased during forced exhalation by the added contraction of the abdominals, as when you are running, to help force air out of the lungs quickly. This action of the abdominals is used in various forms of pranayama that require strong and quick exhalations. The abdominals are not used much during quiet breathing.

EXPERIENTIAL ANATOMY

For Practicing

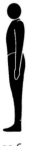

12.6

TADASANA

Applied Practice 1: The Effect of Tadasana on the Excursion of the Diaphragm
Prop: 1 nonskid mat
Take Care: Stand on a level surface.
STAND IN TADASANA on your nonskid mat (Figure 12.6). Make sure that your spine is adjusted so that all your curves are neutral. Now take a deep breath and notice how easy that is to do. Allow your lumbar spine to flex slightly and try to take a deep breath again. Notice that the second breath is much harder to take and feels incomplete. This is because the change in vertebral position affects the normal excursion of the diaphragm. Remember this connection between vertebral position and diaphragmatic freedom, not only in asana practice but throughout your daily activities as well.

Applied Practice 2: Sama Vrtti Pranayama with Rib Movement

Props: 4 or 5 blankets (or 4 blankets and 1 bolster)

       1 nonskid mat • 1 eye bag or eye cover

Take Care: Do not practice this pose if you are more than three months pregnant.

Preparing Blankets:

#1: folded to 2.5" x 10" x 28"

#2: folded to 5" x 7.5" x 28"

#3: folded to 1" x 21" x 28" and rolled firmly from its short end

(or 1 round bolster)

#4: folded as for #1 and then rolled to a final dimension of 5" x 6" x 28"

#5: to cover yourself, for warmth (optional)

PLACE BLANKET #1 in the middle of your nonskid mat so the long sides of the blanket and mat are parallel; place blanket #2 where your head will be. Sit on the mat in Dandasana, with the blankets behind you and with blanket #1 pulled in snugly to touch your buttocks. Lie back and adjust blanket #2 so it supports your entire neck and the back of your head.

After you have made sure that your first two blankets are well arranged, roll to your side, sit up, and place the fatter of the two blanket rolls (or a bolster) under your knees, so that it supports your calves and thighs evenly, and place the thinner roll under your Achilles tendons. Cover up with blanket #5 if you tend to get chilly. Lie down and cover your eyes (Fgure 12.7).

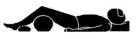

12.7
RECLINING
SAMA VRTTI
PRANAYAMA

Spend the first few minutes relaxing in Savasana: feet falling away from each other, arms out from your sides, palms up. Make sure that your spine is completely and comfortably relaxed, your buttocks are on the floor, and your chest is elevated. Now begin to pay attention to your breath. Just let it be, but be there with it. Gradually begin to lengthen each inhalation and match it with an equal exhalation, so both parts of the breath are *sama,* or even.

Now begin to use your ribs in this manner. As you inhale, focus on lifting your ribs out to the side; as the exhalation follows, let the ribs drop slowly. Try this for 3 to 5 breaths. For the second part of the breath practice, focus on the ribs moving as a whole, gliding upward toward the head on inhalation and slowly moving toward the pelvis on exhalation. Again focus on this rib movement for 3 to 5 breaths. The last series is to imagine your rib cage getting deeper with each inhalation. That is, as you inhale, let your breastbone lift toward the ceiling and your back ribs move toward the floor for 3 to 5 breaths. As you do these three aspects of rib movement, make sure that there is no strain and that your breath is even at all times.

After completing each of these three aspects, try them all at once as you breathe a soft long breath in and an equal soft long breath out. Try this final part for 5 to 20 breaths. When you are finished, let your breathing return to a natural state but observe the residual effects in your lungs, ribs, and muscles. Lie for a few minutes in relaxation before rolling to the side and slowly sitting up.

For Teaching

Applied Teaching 1: Supported Setu Bandhasana to Open the Diaphragm
Props: 2 blankets • 1 nonskid mat
Take Care: Avoid this pose if you suffer from hiatal hernia, are more than three months pregnant, or have concerns about your head being lower than your chest.
Preparing Blankets:
Fold both blankets to measure 5" x 7.5" x 28"

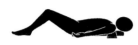

12.8
SUPPORTED
SETU
BANDHASANA

HAVE YOUR STUDENT place one blanket on her nonskid mat so the long sides of the blanket and mat are parallel. Have her position the second blanket across the first so they form a +. Ask her to sit down on the mat, close to the bottom blanket and lie back over the setup. Her buttocks should be on the floor and her entire spine well supported (Figure 12.8).

Make sure that her head is hanging back a bit and her rib cage is lifted. In fact, this position should cause her lower ribs to flare to the sides. Her arms rest opened out to the side. Spend a moment to help your student be comfortable. This, and the opening of the rib cage, is what make this a back bend. Suggest that she stay in the pose for 5 to 10 minutes. She may enjoy some deep breathing in the pose. To come out, suggest that she roll to the side and sit up carefully using her arms.

Applied Teaching 2: Observing the Rib Cage in Sama Vrtti
Props: 4 blankets (or 3 blankets and 1 bolster)
       1 nonskid mat • 1 eye bag or eye cover
Take Care: Do not practice this pose if you are more than three months pregnant.
Preparing Blankets: Fold and roll your blankets as for Applied Practice 2, in this chapter.

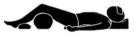

12.9
SAVASANA,
WITH PROPS

HAVE YOUR STUDENT set up as for Practice 2, Sama Vrtti Pranayama, including the cover over the eyes (Figure 12.9). Once he is comfortable, sit by his side and observe his breathing pattern. Observe the three directions of movement: opening of the ribs to the side, then movement of the rib cage as a whole toward the head and back toward the pelvis on exhalation, and the deepening of his rib cage from top to bottom.

Now suggest that he increase the range of movement in each of the areas, one by one. Once he has tried several breaths in all three areas, if there is a specific movement that is limited, have him practice that movement 10 to 15 times more. After 5 to 7 minutes of observation, have him continue on his own for another 5 to 10 minutes. Then he should lie still for 10 more minutes before rolling to his side and sitting up slowly.

Uddiyana bandha is a lock created in part by the diaphragm. The word *uddiyana* means, roughly, "to fly up like a great bird." It should not be practiced by pregnant or menstruating women or until six months postpartum. It is not recommended for those suffering from hypertension or for six months after abdominal surgery.

This bandha is best attempted on an empty stomach, for example, in the morning after evacuation and before breakfast. To practice it, stand up, lean over, and rest your hands on partially bent knees, while keeping your elbows straight.

Drop your head and exhale strongly and completely. Now contract your abdominal muscles as if to draw your belly to your backbone, as you image your lower ribs moving outward slightly. Hold for 3 seconds, then inhale and relax. Repeat several more times. You can practice this bandha at the beginning of your regular asana practice several times a week. It is believed to positively affect the abdominal organs and to move prana, or energy, into the *kunda,* or vessel, of the core body.

PART FIVE
The Upper Extremity

The Shoulder Girdle 13

THE WAY WE carry our shoulders and arms sends a message to the world. Not surprisingly, many common expressions incorporate these messages into our daily conversations: shoulder a burden, shoulder to the wheel, lean on my shoulder, pull your shoulders back, chip on your shoulder, broad shoulders, stoop-shouldered, shouldering responsibility, standing on someone's shoulders, built upon someone's shoulders, looking over your shoulder, carrying the weight of the world on your shoulders, having a good head on your shoulders. These expressions convey a mood, an attitude, a certain level of competence, which we assume by how we carry our shoulders. When we stand with our shoulders open and back, we feel more alive and positive. When we stand with our shoulders drooped and forward, we feel less energetic and sadder.

Arm positions can be as revealing as shoulder positions. Habitually standing with arms crossed over the chest is a way to shut off, separate, and protect oneself. Becoming aware of your habitual shoulder and arm positions (and teaching your students to do the same) will not only improve your asana practice but may improve your life as well, by bringing awareness to this important area.

The shoulder girdle, unlike the pelvic girdle, is constructed more for movement than for stability (Figures 13.1 and 13.2). The pelvic girdle is a solid bony ring, while the shoulder girdle is more loosely joined together. Try this experiment. Whatever position your body is in right now, move one of your hip joints an inch in any direction. You will find that the other hip joint invariably moves. Now try the same experiment with one of your arms. Move one arm around and you will find that the other arm stays still. Of course, the arms are indirectly connected through the scapulae and clavicles, but that connection is much looser than the hips. The shoulder girdle is not designed for bearing weight, as is the pelvic girdle. For this reason

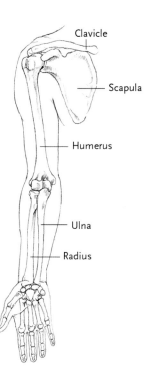

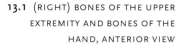

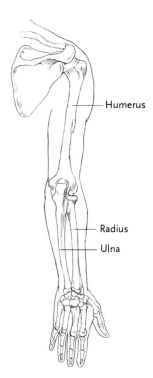

13.1 (RIGHT) BONES OF THE UPPER
EXTREMITY AND BONES OF THE
HAND, ANTERIOR VIEW

13.2 (FAR RIGHT) BONES OF THE
UPPER EXTREMITY AND BONES
OF HAND, POSTERIOR VIEW

alone, understanding the structure and function of the shoulder girdle is important for the teachers and students of yoga who regularly use it for weight bearing in poses such as Salamba Sirsasana, Salamba Sarvangasana, and Adho Mukha Vrksasana. This understanding can help you to prevent injuries to this area of the body.

BONES

For asana practice, the most significant bone of the shoulder girdle is the scapula. Understanding the position of the scapula, how it moves and what muscles make that happen, is imperative if you are to understand the upper extremity in asana. In addition, understanding the need for the scapula to be stabilized well in poses demanding strength is equally important.

The scapula is a triangular-shaped bone that, while curved, sits in an almost vertical position when the student is standing in Tadasana. The important anatomical bony landmarks on the scapula are:

▶ vertebral border (medial side): the long side of the scapula near the vertebral column

▶ axillary border (lateral side): the long side of the scapula on the lateral side near the armpit

▶ inferior angle: the angle located at the base of the bone

▶ spine: on the posterior side of the bone, running almost horizontally from the medial side of the bone, ending in the acromion

▶ acromion: the wide shelf of the scapula which covers the superior gleno-humeral joint

▶ supraspinatus fossa: the hollow on the posterior surface above the spine, which is the origin for the supraspinatus muscle

▶ infraspinatus fossa: the flattened posterior surface inferior to the spine, which is the origin for the infraspinatus muscle

▶ subscapular fossa: the anterior surface of the scapula, which is the origin for the subscapularis

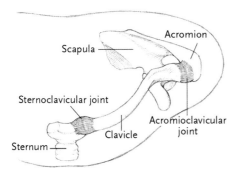

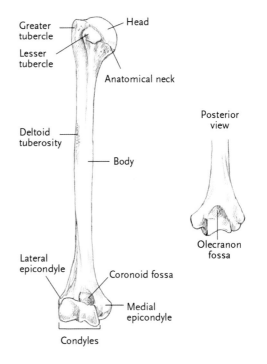

Greater tubercle

Head

Lesser tubercle

Anatomical neck

Deltoid tuberosity

Body

Posterior view

Lateral epicondyle

Coronoid fossa

Olecranon fossa

Medial epicondyle

Condyles

13.3 (ABOVE) ACROMIOCLAVICULAR AND STERNOCLAVICULAR JOINTS

13.4 (RIGHT) HUMERUS

▶ glenoid fossa: the shallow, curved surface on the lateral scapula, which articulates with the head of the humerus to create the shoulder joint proper

▶ coracoid process: or "crow's beak," the curved finger-like projection of the scapula that protrudes anteriorly and can be palpated distal to the clavicle. It is the only portion of the scapula that is anterior; it serves as an attachment site for muscles. (Note: While it is true that the subscapular fossa is on the anterior side of the scapula, it is not on the anterior half of the body. Only the coracoid process is on the anterior half of the body.)

The second bone of the shoulder area is the clavicle, which connects to the sternum at the sternoclavicular joint. It joins the scapula at the acromion, or the acromioclavicular joint (Figure 13.3). The clavicle is convex anteriorly on its medial portion but concave anteriorly on its lateral portion. In other words, the clavicle lies in a gentle S shape when viewed from above.

To feel this shape, place the fingers of your right hand gently over the anterior head of the humerus.

Now move your fingers medially toward the sternum along the body of the clavicle. Note how the clavicle is concave here, with the concavity anterior. At about one-third of the way toward the midline, the clavicle begins to curve out anteriorly as it approaches and joins the sternum. At this point, the clavicle is decidedly convex. The major function of the clavicle is to act as a strut to maintain the width and shape of the shoulder girdle. Without clavicles, your shoulder sockets would come very far forward in the front body and almost touch.

The final bone that forms the shoulder joint is the humerus (Figure 13.4). The important anatomical bony landmarks of the humerus are:

▶ head: the rounded, convex surface which sits in the glenoid fossa of the scapula to create the shoulder joint. The head is overlaid one-third with a thin layer of hyaline cartilage because this joint needs a high degree of mobility.

▶ anatomical neck: the portion of the bone that separates the head from the tubercles

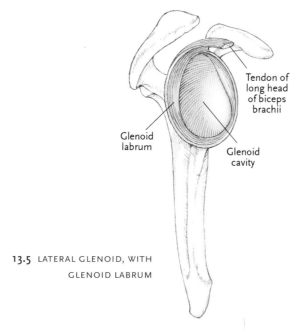

13.5 LATERAL GLENOID, WITH GLENOID LABRUM

▸ greater tubercle: found lateral to the head of the humerus and having three distinct flat impressions, which serve as the insertion points for three shoulder muscles: the supraspinatus, the infraspinatus, and the teres minor

▸ lesser tubercle: projects medially just distal to the neck of the humerus. It serves as the attachment of the subscapularis muscle.

▸ body: the long shaft of the humerus

▸ deltoid tuberosity: the attachment for the deltoid muscle, about halfway down the shaft on the lateral side

▸ condyles: the two distinct rounded medial and lateral structures at the distal humerus that articulate with the radius. The lateral structure is called the capitulum; it articulates with the medial head of the radius when the elbow joint is flexed. The medial condyle of the humerus is called the trochlea; it articulates with the ulna.

▸ lateral epicondyle: a small protruberance on the distal lateral humerus that provides for the attachment of ligaments and muscles

▸ medial epicondyle: a small protruberance on the distal medial humerus above the condyle that provides for the attachment of the ligaments and muscles

▸ coronoid fossa: a depressed hollow area on the anterior distal humerus where the ulna articulates with the humerus during flexion of the elbow

▸ olecranon fossa: a depression on the distal posterior humerus for the ulna to articulate with the humerus during extension of the elbow

JOINTS

The shoulder joint, also called the gleno-humeral joint, is a synovial joint consisting of the articulation of the humeral head with the glenoid fossa of the scapula. Not only do the muscles and ligaments of the joint help hold the humerus in place in the glenoid fossa, but also these elements—ligaments, tendons, and muscles—help maintain the essential integrity of the shoulder capsule. This integrity ensures, in part, the health of the hyaline cartilage by maintaining a watertight compartment so the synovial fluid can provide oxygen and nutrients to the cartilage and thus ensure that various movements of the humeral head are almost frictionless.

Many yoga teachers do not realize that the glenoid fossa of the scapula actually faces approximately 15 degrees anteriorly, as well as laterally and slightly upward (Figure 13.5). This is called anteversion of the shoulder joint. Note the position of the head of the humerus in yourself and in your students during the practice of Tadasana. Pulling the head of the humerus backward to face exactly laterally actually involves external rotation and is not the basic anatomical position.

The glenoid fossa is pear-shaped. Visualize a snowman: the top rounded portion is smaller than the lower rounded portion. The glenoid is similar: the upper, shallower portion allows for smaller movements between the humerus and scapula, and the lower, deeper one allows for larger movements. When movements of the humerus are mainly in the lower portion of the glenoid, they are more stable because there is more congruence between the humerus and glenoid.

The position of maximum stability for the gleno-humeral joint is extension, adduction, and internal rotation of the humerus. This is similar to the position of the gleno-humeral joint in Halasana, with the arms behind the back, especially with the elbows straight and hands interlocked. However, most yoga students externally rotate their shoulder joints in the pose, so they lose one of the components of stability. An example of a position of instability in the upper extremity is hanging over the chair in a supported back bend. Sometimes it is even possible to see the head of the humerus bulging out in the armpit. If this happens, the student should immediately externally rotate the humerus and fully extend the elbow to bring the head of the humerus into a more stable position in the joint. Yoga teachers should be vigilant to make sure students do not habitually overstretch the shoulder joints in this pose, thus contributing to serious hypermobility and possible injury.

The position of most instability for the gleno-humeral joint is flexion, abduction, and external rotation of the humerus. In this position the head of the humerus is moved forward into the upper and shallower portion of the glenoid and is moved anteriorly, to where the ligaments around the joint are less strong. An additional instability factor is that there are few muscles on the anterior shoulder joint that can lend stability to the area.

The acromioclavicular joint is a gliding joint made up of the medial acromion and the lateral end of the clavicle. There is some rotation at this joint during flexion and abduction of the shoulder joint.

The sternocavicular joint consists of the sternal end of the clavicle, the lateral manubrium, and the cartilage of the first rib. This articulation allows very limited movement in most directions.

The final joint of the shoulder area is the scapulo-thoracic joint. This is the articulation of the scapula over the posterior rib cage; whenever the scapula moves, it does so over the bones of the rib cage. In fact, the scapula slides over the ribs on a "bed" of fascia and adipose tissue, which serves as a cushion for the rib cage during scapular movements.

CONNECTIVE TISSUE

The ligaments of the gleno-humeral joint do not function well to keep the bones together; at this joint, they mainly function to limit movement.

The main ligaments of the gleno-humeral joint are:

▶ articular capsule: This completely encircles the joint and is attached outside the glenoid labrum and to the neck of the humerus. The gleno-humeral ligaments are incorporated in the capsule itself. The head of the humerus is about three times bigger than the glenoid fossa, so the ligaments are very important for stabilization of the shoulder joint (Figure 13.6).

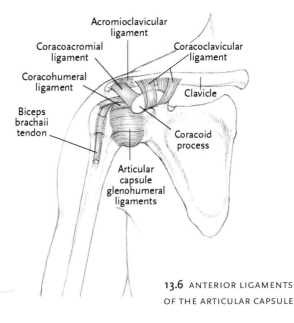

Acromioclavicular ligament
Coracoacromial ligament
Coracoclavicular ligament
Coracohumeral ligament
Clavicle
Biceps brachaii tendon
Coracoid process
Articular capsule glenohumeral ligaments

13.6 ANTERIOR LIGAMENTS OF THE ARTICULAR CAPSULE

The capsule is pierced by the tendon of the long head of the biceps brachii. The capsule folds and covers the biceps tendon into the intertubular groove of the humerus.

It is important to note that the humerus bone hangs loosely in a dependent position in the capsule in Tadasana. Thus the upper portion of the capsule is stretched taut, and the inferior portion is loose and pleated at the axillary fold (armpit). The opposite occurs in full abduction. Here the superior capsule is lax, and the axillary portion is taut.

To better visualize the state of the capsule, look at the top of your student's sleeve in Tadasana. In this pose, the top of the sleeve will be taut. When she raises her arm overhead, the top of the sleeve bunches, and the fabric at the bottom of the armpit is stretched taut. The capsule of the shoulder joint is the same. When the humerus is in a recumbent position, the top of the capsule is stretched; when the humerus is in full flexion, the bottom of the capsule is stretched. When she abducts her humerus to perform Vrksasana, however, holding her arm over her head, the opposite is true. In full abduction, the top of her sleeve is loose and bunched, and the axillary portion is stretched. So is the capsule.

With the humerus in the dependent position of Tadasana, the superior tautness helps to prevent the downward dislocation of the humerus. The superior laxity of the capsule that is created during abduction helps make this motion possible. Remember the superior laxity of the capsule during abduction. Because of this laxity, there is the possibility of impingement of the superior capsule between the humerus and the acromion during abduction, which can cause pain and inflammation and can contribute to a decrease of normal function in the shoulder joint. An example of an asana in which this can happen is when your student raises her arms over her head to practice Vrksasana.

▶ glenoid labrum: The word *labrum* means "lip." The glenoid labrum is a fibrocartilaginous ring on the perimeter of the glenoid fossa that helps to create a deeper shoulder joint socket.

In contrast, the acetabulum is created by a much deeper bony indentation in the pelvis. While the depth of the shoulder socket is increased by the glenoid labrum, it is nonetheless much less stable than the hip joint.

The shoulder joint is further supported by the glenohumeral ligaments, which are the main ligaments of the joint. These are three in number: the superior, the inferior, and the medial glenohumeral ligaments. These ligaments thicken the anterior portion of the joint.

Other important ligaments (Figures 13.6 and 13.7) that help to reinforce the shoulder joint include:

▶ acromioclavicular ligament: runs from the acromion to the clavicle

▶ coracoclavicular ligament: runs from the acromion to the coracoid process

▶ coracoacromial ligament: attaches from the acromion to the coracoid process

▶ coracohumeral ligament: covers and reinforces the upper part of the capsule and is attached from the coracoid process to the greater tubercle of the humerus

▶ sternoclavicular ligament: has an anterior and posterior portion that connects the sternum and the clavicle

▶ costoclavicular ligament: runs from the superior first rib to the inferior surface of the first rib

The shoulder joint is surrounded by bursae to protect the tendons of shoulder muscles from too much wear and tear around the joint. These include:

▶ subdeltoid bursa: located between the deltoid muscle and the humerus

▶ subacromial bursa: located between the acromion and the capsule of the shoulder joint

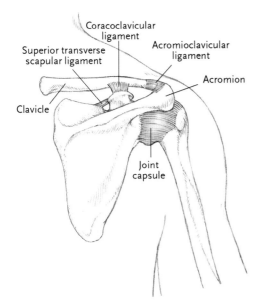

13.7 POSTERIOR/SUPERIOR LIGAMENTS OF THE SHOULDER CAPSULE

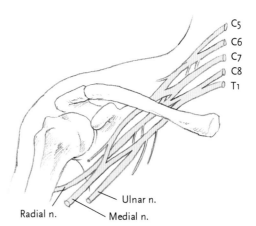

13.8 BRACHIAL PLEXUS

► subcoracoid bursa: located between the coracoid and the shoulder capsule

► coracobrachialis bursa: located between the coracoid and the coracobrachialis

► infraspinatus bursa: located between the tendon of the infraspinatus and the capsule

► others: bursae between the tendons of the latisimus dorsi and the humerus, the teres major and the humerus, and the pectoralis major and the humerus

NERVES

The nerves to the upper extremity are a complex structure called the brachial plexus. It is formed by nerve roots from C5 to T1, which give rise to many branches that innervate the shoulder muscles. These nerves course distally down the arm and forearm, eventually forming the radial, medial, and ulnar nerves (Figure 13.8).

It is important for yoga teachers to be aware of all the origins of the nerves of the brachial plexus

in order to be able to recognize signs of irritation to the plexus if it manifests during asana practice. Any numbness, tingling, or radiating pain in the student's arm or hand should be cause for concern. If it continues beyond a few minutes, the student should seek the counsel of a qualified health practitioner.

If you are not experiencing any problems with the nerves of your brachial plexus, there is a simple way to feel what overstretching these nerves feels like. Either standing or sitting, stretch your right arm out in abduction, about half way up to full abduction. Now extend your wrist strongly, and turn your head as far as you can away from your wrist. This should put some traction on the nerves of your right brachial plexus and create a slightly uncomfortable feeling along the pathway of the nerves. Do this only for a moment, to feel the stretch.

Pressure on the nerves of the brachial plexus is sometimes felt by students during the practice of Salamba Sarvangasana. A common example is when students with tight shoulders attempt to hold the back in the pose and state that their hands are feeling a tingling sensation or are going numb.

If this happens, it is not immediately obvious if the compression on the nerves is coming from the student's neck or from the brachial plexus. Here's how to find out. Have your student practice Salamba Sarvangasana with his feet on the wall, so his tibias are parallel to the floor and his back is straight. Now ask him to remove his hands from his back and stretch out his arms to the side. Make sure he keeps his feet on the wall for balance. If the tingling is relieved almost immediately, it is likely that the compression of the brachial plexus nerves as they pass through this axillary area has been relieved.

MUSCLES

The muscles of the shoulder joint are myriad, and their interactions are complex. In order to fully understand the movements at the gleno-humeral and related joints, it is strongly recommend that you memorize the origins, insertions, and actions of all the following muscles: the muscles that connect the scapula to the vertebral column (Figures 13. 9 and 13.10), the muscles that connect the upper limb to the trunk (Figures 13.11 and 13.12), and the muscles of the shoulder joint proper (Figures 13.13a, 13.13b, 13.13c, 13.14, and 13.15).

KINESIOLOGY

A little-appreciated aspect of the kinesiology of the biceps brachii muscle can be helpful to yoga teachers when they are assisting students. Most of us think of the primary action of the biceps muscle as being elbow flexion, and indeed it is. It is the muscle most often used to show "muscle man" strength. The biceps is also a shoulder flexor. But the strongest action performed by the biceps brachii is supination of the forearm.

In order to experience this, sit with your ver-

tebral column in its natural curves, with your right shoulder joint in about 45 degrees of flexion and your elbow joint in 90 degrees of flexion and pronated. Now lightly palpate your right biceps brachii muscle as you flex your elbow against an imaginary force.

Notice the amount of force you generate in your biceps as you flex your elbow joint. Now try it again, and this time as your flex your elbow, gradually supinate your forearm, again against a strong imaginary force. You will feel a greatly increased amount of force of contraction in your biceps when you are supinating while flexing, as compared with flexion and pronation.

In fact, the biceps brachii's greatest action is to act as a supinator. Therefore, if you want to maximize the strength of your biceps as an elbow or shoulder flexor, always flex your elbow and shoulder joint in supination. Placing your forearm in supination, with your palms up, will allow you a stronger mechanical advantage as a teacher when you perform an aid like pulling back on a strap in poses like Adho Mukha Svanasana or when pulling with a pole to help your student stretch her shoulders. And if you want to perform the classic callisthenic movement of a pull-up, it will be easier in supination because your biceps will have the greatest mechanical advantage as an elbow and shoulder flexor with your elbow joint in supination.

THE GLENO-HUMERAL RHYTHM

The most significant aspect of movement in the shoulder joint is the gleno-humeral rhythm. This rhythm is a special action around the shoulder joint which involves the scapula, humerus, and clavicle in a rhythmic way. The gleno-humeral rhythm accompanies the shoulder movements of flexion and abduction. If the rhythm is disturbed by injury, pathological process, or weakness, the result can be pain and a reduction in healthy movement.

The easiest way to learn the gleno-humeral

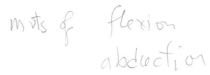
mvts of flexion
abduction

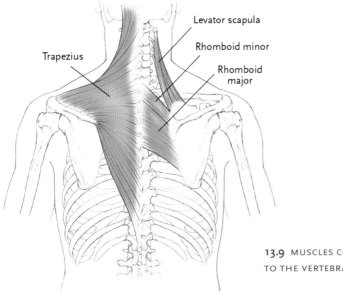

13.9 MUSCLES CONNECTING THE SCAPULA
TO THE VERTEBRAL COLUMN

13.10   MUSCLES CONNECTING THE SCAPULA TO THE VERTEBRAL COLUMN

MUSCLE	ORIGIN	INSERTION	ACTION
Trapezius	External occipital protuberance; ligamentum nuchae; middle ⅓ of nuchal line of occipital bone; spinous processes of C7 and T1-T12; supraspinal ligament	Superior fibers: lateral ⅓ of clavicle; Middle fibers: medial acromium and spine of scapula	Rotates, adducts scapula; upper fibers elevate scapula; lower fibers depress scapula
Rhomboid major	Spinous processes of T2, T3, T4, and T5; supraspinal ligament	Spine of scapula; inferior angle of scapula	Adducts scapula
Rhomboid minor	Ligamentun nuchae; spinous processes of C7 and T1	Spine of scapula	Adducts scapula
Levator scapula	Transverse processes of C1, C2, C3, and C4	Vertebral border of scapula	Elevates scapula; with scapula fixed, side bends cervical spine and rotates it toward same side

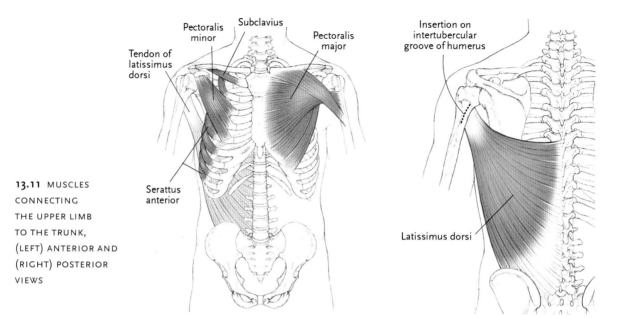

13.11 MUSCLES CONNECTING THE UPPER LIMB TO THE TRUNK, (LEFT) ANTERIOR AND (RIGHT) POSTERIOR VIEWS

Labels (left, anterior view): Pectoralis minor · Subclavius · Pectoralis major · Tendon of latissimus dorsi · Serattus anterior

Labels (right, posterior view): Insertion on intertubercular groove of humerus · Latissimus dorsi

13.12   MUSCLES CONNECTING THE UPPER LIMBS TO THE TRUNK

MUSCLE	ORIGIN	INSERTION	ACTION
Pectoralis major	Medial half of sternum; anterior sternum; cartilages of all true ribs except 1 and 7; aponeurosis of external oblique	Greater tubercle of humerus	Flexes, adducts, and medially rotates humerus
Pectoralis minor	Superior margins of ribs 3, 4, and 5	Coracoid process	Elevates and depresses scapula; raises ribs 3, 4, and 5 in forced inhalation
Subclavius	Rib 1	Inferior clavicle	Elevates shoulder
Serratus anterior	Superior border of ribs 1–9	Anterior surface of vertebral border of scapula	Rotates scapula for full flexion and abduction; protracts scapula
Latissimus dorsi	Thoraco–lumbar fascia; lower 6 thoracic and all lumbar and sacral vertebrae; supraspinal ligament; posterior crest of ilium	Intertubercular groove of humerus	Extends, adducts, and rotates arm medially; draws shoulder downward and backward

rhythm is to remember that it involves four muscles, four bones, and four movements. The four muscles are called either the rotator cuff muscles, or equally often, the SITS muscles, for the first letter of each muscle's name (Figure 13.16). The SITS muscles, charted in Figure 13.15, are the supraspinatus, infraspinatus, subscapularis, and teres minor.

The four bones are the scapula, the humerus, the clavicle, and the thoracic spine. (The thoracic spine actually consists of twelve bones, but for the ease of learning the gleno-humeral rhythm, we will count it as one bone.) Here's how the gleno-humeral rhythm works. The four SITS contract in a specific overlapping order to create the smooth movements of flexion and abduction. The bones are moved in the following way: the scapula protracts, and the glenoid is rotated cranially; the head of the humerus is cinched into the joint, descends to the part of the glenoid that is deeper and larger, and externally rotates; the clavicle rotates longitudinally inward toward the chest cavity; and the thoracic spine extends. When all these actions are coordinated perfectly, you are able to flex and abduct your shoulder joint normally.

To have a clearer experience of the external rotation component of the gleno-humeral rhythm, try this. While sitting or standing, place one hand over the anterior surface of your other arm, about midway between the elbow and the shoulder joint. Now perform flexion with the straight arm, and feel the external rotation that occurs under your hand. Try it again on the other side. External rotation of the humerus is a key movement of both flexion and abduction of the shoulder joint.

The longitudinal rotation of your clavicle can be felt by placing your index and middle finger tips on either side of the opposite clavicle. Find the place where the clavicle is rounded out, just lateral to its articulation with the sternum. Lightly but firmly hold the bone between your fingers while you abduct that arm. You will feel your clavicle rotating inward, back, and down as you abduct. This rotation is a necessary part of the gleno-humeral rhythm and helps allow the scapula to move as it needs to for full abduction and flexion.

STABILIZATION

After the gleno-humeral rhythm, the other important kinesiological principle necessary to understand the shoulder joint is stabilization. The ability to practice poses requiring strength from the shoulder joint depends on stabilization of the scapula. This means that the scapula is held stable against the rib cage in a neutral position. This requires the action of the intrascapular muscles like the middle trapezius, the rhomboids, and the serratus anterior.

Here is a simple way to feel the importance of stabilization. Sitting or standing, flex your shoulder joints to 90 degrees, and extend your wrists so you are looking at the back of your hands. Now let your scapulae protract. Next pretend that you are pushing away an elephant. Really use your muscles as if you were actually doing this task. You will find that you do not have much power in this movement.

Keeping your arms in flexion, draw your scapulae down and slightly together so they are in a neutral position and held firmly against your rib cage. Now push outward, as if you are pushing the imaginary elephant. You will notice a great increase in the power you experience in this movement.

Stabilizing the scapulae against the rib cage in a neutral position keeps the glenoid in a neutral position and thus facilitates the maximum power of all the shoulder muscles. Remember to suggest that your students place their scapulae in neutral for such strength poses as Chaturanga Dandasana and Adho Mukha Vrksasana.

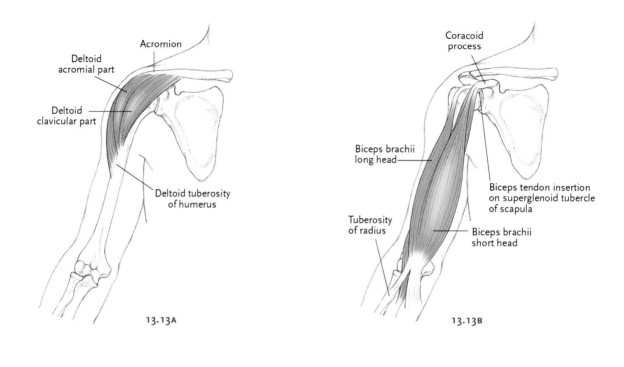

13.13A

13.13B

13.13C

13.14

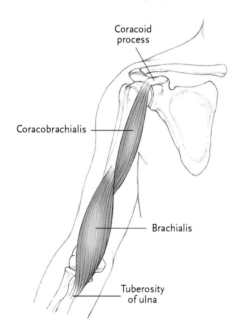

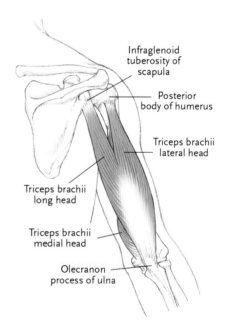

13.13A, B, AND C MUSCLES OF THE UPPER EXTREMITY, ANTERIOR VIEW

13.14 MUSCLES OF THE SHOULDER JOINT, POSTERIOR VIEW

MUSCLE	ORIGIN	INSERTION	ACTION
Deltoid	Anterior: lateral ⅓ of clavicle; middle: lateral acromion; posterior: spine of the scapula	Deltoid tuberosity of humerus	Anterior: flexes, horizontally adducts, medially rotates humerus; middle: abducts humerus to 90 degrees; posterior: extends, externally rotates, horizontally abducts
Subscapularis	Subscapular fossa	Lesser tubercle of humerus	Internally rotates humerus
Supraspinatus	Supraspinatus fossa	Highest point of greater tubercle of humerus	Abducts shoulder joint and draws humerus into glenoid; stabilizes
Infraspinatus	Infraspinatus fossa	Middle impression of greater tubercle of humerus	Rotates shoulder joint externally
Teres minor	Cranial ⅔ of axillary border of scapula	Lowest impression of greater tubercle of humerus	Rotates shoulder joint externally
Teres major	Posterior surface of inferior angle of scapula	Lesser tubercle of anterior humerus	Internally rotates and adducts humerus
Coracobrachialis	Coracoid process of scapula	Medial body of humerus	Flexes and adducts humerus
Biceps brachii, short head	Coracoid process of scapula	Tuberosity of radius	Flexes shoulder joint, flexes elbow, and supinates forearm
Biceps brachii, long head	Supraglenoid tubercle of scapula	Tuberosity of radius and bicipital aponeurosis	Flexes shoulder joint, flexes elbow, and supinates forearm
Brachialis	Distal anterior humerus	Tuberosity of ulna and coracoid process	Flexes elbow
Triceps brachii, long head	Infraglenoid tuberosity of scapula	Olecranon process of ulna	Extends shoulder joint and elbow
Triceps brachii, medial head	Posterior body of humerus	Olecranon process of ulna	Extends elbow
Triceps brachii, lateral head	Posterior body of humerus	Olecranon process of ulna	Extends elbow

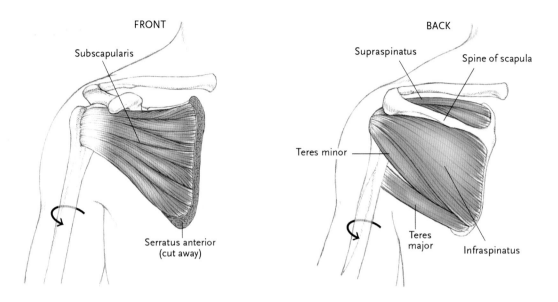

FRONT

Subscapularis

Serratus anterior
(cut away)

BACK

Supraspinatus

Spine of scapula

Teres minor

Teres
major

Infraspinatus

13.16 ROTATOR CUFF MUSCLES: SUPRASPINATUS, INFRASPINATUS, TERES MINOR, AND SUBSCAPULARIS

SPECIFIC SHOULDER PROBLEMS

The shoulder joint is prone to a number of problems that range from annoying to serious. They include:

▶ dislocation: when the head of the humerus is pulled out of the glenoid fossa. It is both very painful and very serious and requires immediate medical aid.

▶ shoulder separation: when the clavicle is forcefully separated from the scapula at the acromio-clavicular joint. This separation usually occurs in athletic injuries when the individual falls on the top of the shoulder. It requires immediate medical aid.

▶ bursitis: the irritation and inflammation of the bursal sac of the shoulder. Bursitis is a secondary condition created by a primary problem with the biomechanical function of the rotator cuff. It is usually caused when the head of the humerus does not move down in the glenoid during abduction, so the greater tuberosity presses up against the

subacromial bursa. This can occur in any pose in which the arm is repeatedly abducted and sometimes by repeated flexion. Bursitis of the shoulder joint can also occur at the subdeltoid bursa. It usually occurs after a sudden unguarded movement or after unusually long repetitive movements.

▶ tendonitis: an irritation to a tendon. The most common forms of tendonitis in the shoulder joint are to the suprascapular, or long head of the biceps tendon.

▶ frozen shoulder: an effect of a long-lasting dysfunction of the gleno-humeral rhythm, causing the shoulder to be used less. A downward spiral is created by an initial injury that creates pain, which leads to less movement, which leads to more pain and guarding. Eventually movement can become less painful but more and more restricted, until the shoulder joint is referred to as frozen.

The three stages of a frozen shoulder are:
stage one: The individual can lie on the involved side on that shoulder, does not have pain to the wrist, has no pain at night. When tested by a

trained professional, the joint will exhibit an elastic passive joint movement with a limitation of movement of only 20 to 30 degrees. Pain is only felt on extreme movement.

stage two: The individual can still lie on the involved side, does not have pain to the wrist, but does have pain either in the day with extreme movements and/or at night at rest.

stage three: The individual cannot lie on the involved side, has pain to the wrist, the shoulder hurts at night only, the capsule has lost all elastic passive movement, and there is an extreme capsular limitation. The least limited movement is internal rotation, then abduction, with external rotation being the most limited. The individual needs to be under the care of a physical therapist or other knowledgable health care professional and should not attend asana classes until movement improves.

EXPERIENTIAL ANATOMY

For Practicing

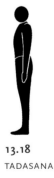

13.17
TADASANA,
WITH THE
HAND ON
THE SHOULDER

Applied Practice 1: Feeling the Rotational Movement of the Humerus in Abduction
Prop: 1 nonskid mat
Take Care: Avoid this practice if you have pain on abduction.

To FEEL the rotational movement of your humerus during abduction, sit or stand with your feet on your mat and normal spinal curves in place, and then place your left fingertips across the upper outer portion of your right shoulder, where your sleeve begins (Figure 13.17). Abduct your right humerus at a moderate speed. Notice the spontaneous external rotation that begins after about 30 degrees of movement. Try it on both sides to see if there is any difference.

13.18
TADASANA

Applied Practice 2: Feeling the Effect of No Rotation of the Humerus on Full Abduction
Prop: 1 nonskid mat
Take Care: Avoid this practice if you have pain on abduction.

To FEEL the external rotation component in abduction, begin by sitting or standing on your nonskid mat, with all the curves of your vertebral column in neutral (Figure 13.18). Now internally rotate your left humerus and, while keeping it internally rotated, try to abduct it. You will be unable to do it, as the head of the humerus will hit against the shelf of the acromion and stop the movement of abduction. Start again in internal rotation, but this time when you feel the bony block occur, immediately externally rotate the humerus and let it swing out under the shelf of the acromion, thus permitting full abduction.

For Teaching

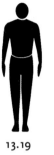

13.19
TADASANA

Applied Teaching 1: Palpating the Shoulder Area

Prop: 1 nonskid mat

Take Care: Be sure to ask for your student's permission before touching her.

HAVE HER STAND in Tadasana on a nonskid mat (Figure 13.19). Standing in front of the student, gently trace the clavicle from the sternum to the acromion. Then palpate the coracoid process under the lateral clavicle. Now walk around behind her and trace gently the vertebral border and axillary border of the bone. You may need to ask your student to abduct her humerus to at least 90 degrees in order to do this latter palpation. Now trace the spine of the scapula from its medial border to the acromion. Finally, locate the inferior angle.

13.20
TADASANA

Applied Teaching 2: Observing Gleno-Humeral Rhythm

Prop: 1 nonskid mat

Take Care: Avoid these movements if they produce pain.

ASK YOUR STUDENT to stand in Tadasana on a nonskid mat (Figure 13.20). Stand behind him. It is helpful if his clothing allows for an easy viewing of his scapula. Ask him to abduct both his humerus bones from neutral to full abduction several times in a row, at a moderate speed. Note the rhythmic movement of the scapulae as he does so. Now have him flex from neutral to full flexion, and again observe the scapular movements. One interesting variation of this observation is to have him abduct one extremity and flex the other, and note that the end point of both of these actions is the same. You can even have him do the movements while your eyes are closed. Upon the completion of the movements, open your eyes and try to guess which extremity was abducted and which was flexed.

Applied Teaching 3: Observing the Gleno-Humeral Rhythm in Adho Mukha Svanasana

Prop: 1 nonskid mat

Take Care: Avoid these movements if they cause pain in the shoulder joint.

ONE OF THE most commonly practiced poses to stretch the shoulder joint is Adho Mukha Svanasana (Figure 13.21). Have your students practice this pose on a nonskid mat and observe their shoulder joint movement. Remember that in order to obtain full flexion of the shoulder joint, we need to externally rotate the humerus as well.

13.21
ADHO MUKHA
SVANASANA

However, if at the full range of shoulder flexion in Adho Mukha Svanasana the student continues to externally rotate, she will actually begin to limit her movement. Beginning students do well to focus on allowing external rotation to naturally occur as they come into the pose. But once the full flexion is just about reached, have your experienced student internally rotate instead. This will actually create more freedom in her shoulder joint.

You can experience this first before teaching it by doing the following. Sit or stand with your vertebral column in its neutral curves. Then fully flex one shoulder joint; notice how the humerus externally rotates as you do so. At the end of the movement, try to continue externally rotating. It will feel as if the humerus is dropping into the glenoid and that there is actually less freedom if you attempt to flex more. Now do the opposite: at the end of flexion, begin to internally rotate. Paradoxically you will experience more freedom to fully flex at this point. To review, external rotation of the humerus in the glenoid is absolutely necessary for normal and full flexion. However, for yoga students who are close to being at the full range of flexion, try teaching them internal rotation as they settle into Adho Mukha Svanasana.

Applied Teaching 4: Strengthening the Shoulder Muscles

Prop: 1 nonskid mat

Take Care: Avoid these movements if they cause discomfort in the shoulder joint.

AN EFFECTIVE MOVEMENT you can offer students to strengthen the muscles around the shoulder joint is a movement based on preparation for Salamba Sirsasana (Figure 13.22). This movement will strengthen the rotator cuff muscles, the chest muscles, and the muscles of the back and abdomen.

Have your student get down on his hands and knees on a nonskid mat, interlock his fingers as for Salamba Sirsasana, and then lift his hips by straightening his knees. He should then move forward with an exhalation as if to place his body into a straight line over his hands (Figure 13.23). He then moves backward to create the inverted V shape again (Figure 13.22). Be sure that he keeps his elbows on the floor and the breath moving with each back-and-forward movement. Have him practice these movements for 5 to 10 repetitions, exhaling as he moves forward and inhaling as he moves backward.

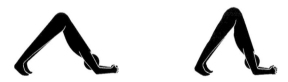

13.22 + 13.23
ARDHA
SALAMBA
SIRSASANA

After a brief rest, have him reverse the interlock of his fingers so that the opposite thumb is on top and all the fingers fit together one slot over, and repeat the movements. To make the movement easier, have him move his feet back, widening the distance between elbows and feet. To make it more challenging, have him move his feet closer to his elbows.

Applied Teaching 5: Stabilizing the Scapula in Chaturanga Dandasana

Prop: 1 nonskid mat

Take Care: Avoid this practice if it causes pain in the shoulder area and during menstruation, pregnancy, and for three months postpartum.

HAVE THE STUDENT spread her nonskid mat on a level surface and practice Chaturanga Dandasana by first coming into a plank position and then lowering into the pose (Figures 13.24 and 13.25).

To avoid injury to the shoulder in Chaturanga Dandasana, the keys are the positions of the scapula and the humerus. Remember, the scapula is the core stabilizing bone of the shoulder joint. To keep the shoulder joint safe in this pose, make sure that the scapulae are held down toward the waist as well as slightly adducted, especially at their lower tips.

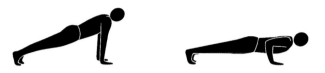

13.24 + 13.25
PLANK POSE +
CHATURANGA
DANDASANA

Additional protection for the shoulder joint in Chaturanga Dandasana can come from paying attention to the position of the top of the humerus bone. Make sure that it is pulled firmly down toward the waist and is externally rotated, elbows close to the body. The top of the humerus bone needs to roll back and downward toward the waist, and at the same time the elbows press downward toward the floor. These two actions of stabilizing the scapula in neutral and descending and externally rotating the head of the humerus in the glenoid decrease the chances of injury.

LINK

A simple and helpful book for rehabilitating the rotator cuff muscles is *The 7-Minute Rotator Cuff Solution: A Complete Program to Prevent and Rehabil-* *itate Rotator Cuff Injuries* by Joseph Horrigan, D.C., and Jerry Robinson (Los Angeles: Health for Life, 1991).

The Elbow Joint and Forearm

PATCH UP THINE OLD BODY FOR HEAVEN.

—DOLL TEARSHEET, IN *KING HENRY IV, PART 2*, BY WILLIAM SHAKESPEARE

MANY STUDENTS COME to asana class having never stood on their hands, and it is a revelation when they learn to do it. For others, standing upside down on the hands or forearms is empowering and fun, recreating the freedom of childhood. But the forearms, wrists, and hands need special attention when they are used for weight bearing in order to protect against injury. Begin cultivating that attention now by learning more about the structures of the area.

BONES

The elbow joint is made up of the humerus (discussed in chapter 13), the ulna, and the radius (Figures 14.1 and 14.2). The ulna is located on the medial side of the forearm. At its proximal posterior end, it forms a point called the olecranon process, which can be felt on the skin as the point of the elbow. When the elbow joint is extended, the curved olecranon glides into the olecranon fossa of the posterior humerus bone.

On the anterior proximal end of the ulna is the coronoid process, which articulates with the coronoid fossa of the anterior humerus on flexion of the elbow joint.

Between the olecranon process and the coronoid process is the trochlear fossa, which is the site of the articulation with the trochlea of the humerus on extension of the joint.

The ulna has a long shaft. At the distal end of the bone are two eminences. The lateral one is termed the head of the ulna, even though it is at the distal end; it articulates with the ulnar notch of the radius. The distal end of the ulna does not articulate directly with the wrist but rather with a fibrocartilage disc that separates it from the carpal bones. The medial eminence is the styloid process.

The radius is so called because during pronation it radiates over the ulna. Regardless of the position of the forearm, the radius bone is on the thumb

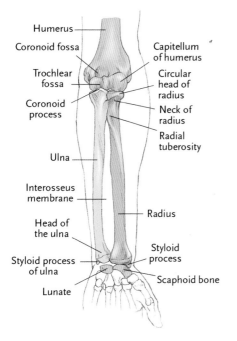

14.1 ELBOW JOINT, ANTERIOR VIEW

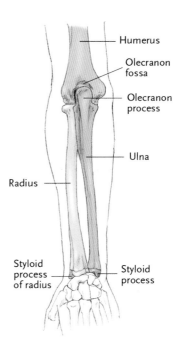

14.2 ELBOW JOINT, POSTERIOR VIEW

side. The radius at its proximal end articulates with the capitulum of the humerus at its structure called the circular head of the radius.

Just below this structure is the neck of the radius, and below that on the medial side is the radial tuberosity, a roughened surface for the attachment of the biceps brachii muscle. On the anterior side is a bursa that pads the tendon of the biceps from the bone.

The distal end of the radius has two articular surfaces. The articular surface on the medial side articulates with the ulna. The other articular surface is on the underside or distal surface of the radius. It serves to articulate with two carpals: the lunate and the scaphoid. The lateral surface of the distal radius is elongated into a prominent process called the styloid process. The process limits radial deviation on the lateral side.

The ulna and the radius are held in place in part by a specific connective tissue called the interosseous membrane. For more information, see the Connective Tissue section in this chapter.

To understand the effect the radial styloid pro-

cess has on movement at the wrist, try this. Place your palm up, about 18 inches from your face, with a slightly abducted shoulder joint. Now flex your wrist, bringing it toward your face. Notice how the medial or ulnar side flexes more, and the radial (thumb) side is able to flex less. This is because the radial styloid process is long and interferes with flexion on the thumb side.

Start in the same position, and attempt radial deviation. This is the movement of trying to bring your thumb toward the radius. Next try the movement in the other direction, toward the ulna. Note how much more freedom there is in ulnar deviation. Again, radial deviation is limited by the length of the radial styloid process.

JOINTS

The elbow joint is actually made up of three different joints. These are the ulnar-humeral, the radio-humeral, and the radio-ulnar joints. The ulnar-humeral joint is a hinge joint, and thus only flexion and extension occur there (Figure 14.3). Because of

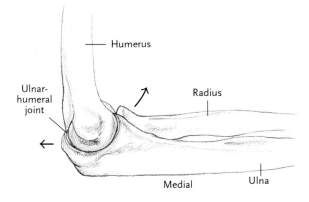

14.3 ULNAR-HUMERAL JOINT

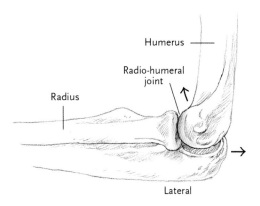

14.4A RADIO-HUMERAL JOINT

joint structure, no lateral movement of any kind is allowed at that joint.

The radio-humeral joint is a gliding joint and very shallow (Figure 14.4a). The joint is held in place by an annular ligament (see Connective Tissue in this chapter). Flexion and extension occur at this joint as well. Flexion is limited at this joint by surrounding soft tissue. However, pronation and supination are free, in part because in these motions the joint surfaces have deep congruence. In other words, a large portion of the joint surfaces of the radius and humerus are fitted together in pronation and supination, thus contributing to the stability of this joint during movement.

The radio-ulnar joint is a pivot joint that allows the radius to radiate, or pivot, over the ulna (Figure 14.4b). The head of the radius is held by the annular ligament against the radial notch on the lateral ulna. This is the point where the radius rotates over the ulna during pronation and supination.

CONNECTIVE TISSUE

Two of the most important ligaments of the elbow joint are the radial and ulnar collateral ligaments. They support the connection of the radius to the humerus and the ulna to the humerus, respectively. The elbow capsule originates around the distal humerus and attaches around the proximal

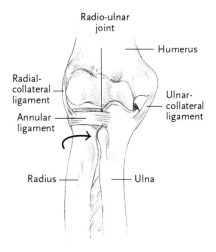

14.4B RADIO-ULNAR JOINT

ulna. The annular and collateral ligaments help to reinforce the capsule.

The annular ligament connects the head of the radius to the radial notch of the ulna on the lateral proximal ulna and serves to prevent the separation of the radius and the humerus in a lateral direction. The interosseus membrane connects nearly the entire line of the ulnar and radial shaft by broad flat fibers. Its fibers are oblique and downward from the radius to the ulna. Not only does this membrane connect the bones; it also allows for the attachment of deep muscles.

For a detailed discussion of the additional ligaments of this area, please consult *Gray's Anatomy*.

NERVES

The nerves of the elbow and forearm are the median, the musculocutaneous, the ulnar, and the radial nerves. The elbow joint proper is innervated by small branches from the ulnar, median, and musculocutaneous nerves. Figure 14.5 illustrates the paths these nerves take down the arm, forearm, and into the hand. Of special note at the elbow joint is the ulnar nerve. This nerve passes distally down the medial side of the arm. As it passes the elbow area, it is found in the groove between the olecranon and the medial epicondyle of the humerus. Because it is very near the surface here, with only a skin and fascial covering, the exposed nerve itself is occasionally hit—what we call hitting the funny bone.

MUSCLES

The muscles of the arm and forearm are a complex group of muscles. The entire first group, which are the superficial flexors, arise from the medial epicondyle of the humerus by a common tendon (Figures 14.6 and 14.7). These muscles on the medial surface of the forearm can be thought of as the flexors of the wrist and hand. Asana and adjustments that require flexion of the wrist require a strong group of flexor muscles. The next group of muscles is deep to the previous one but is still in the flexor group (Figures 14.8 and 14.9).

On the posterior side of the forearm is another group of forearm muscles. The superficial group originates from the lateral supracondylar ridge of the humerus and is part of the extensor group of muscles of the forearm (Figures 14.10 and 14.11). The final and deep group of extensors is listed in Figures 14.12 and 14.13.

KINESIOLOGY

One of the most common positional faults of the elbow joint can become apparent when students take up the practice of yoga asana. It is called hyperextension of the elbow, and it refers specifically to the relationship between the humerus and the ulna on extension of the joint. Normally this angle is approximately 180 degrees. Hyperexten-

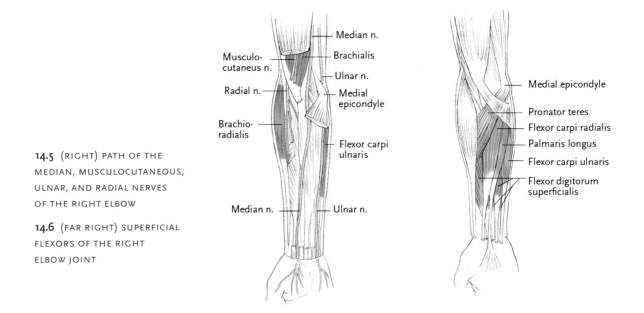

14.5 (RIGHT) PATH OF THE MEDIAN, MUSCULOCUTANEOUS, ULNAR, AND RADIAL NERVES OF THE RIGHT ELBOW

14.6 (FAR RIGHT) SUPERFICIAL FLEXORS OF THE RIGHT ELBOW JOINT

Musculo-cutaneus n.
Radial n.
Brachio-radialis
Median n.

Median n.
Brachialis
Ulnar n.
Medial epicondyle
Flexor carpi ulnaris
Ulnar n.

Medial epicondyle
Pronator teres
Flexor carpi radialis
Palmaris longus
Flexor carpi ulnaris
Flexor digitorum superficialis

MUSCLE	ORIGIN	INSERTION	ACTION
Pronator teres	Humeral head: common flexor tendon, intermuscular septum, medial condyle; ulnar head: coronoid process	Lateral shaft of radius	Pronates forearm (rotating radius on ulna); flexes forearm at elbow
Flexor carpi radialis	Medial epicondyle of humerus	Base of second metacarpal bone	Flexes and abducts wrist
Palmaris longus	Medial epicondyle of humerus	Palmar aponeurosis; flexor retinaculum	Flexes wrist
Flexor carpi ulnaris	Humeral head: medial epicondyle; ulnar head: proximal posterior ulna and olecranon	Pisiform, hamate, and fifth metacarpal	Flexes and adducts wrist
Flexor digitorum superficialis	Medial head: epicondyle of humerus; ulnar head: coronoid process; radial head: anterior oblique line	Middle of second phalanx; base of sides of shaft of middle phalanges of four fingers	Flexes second phalanx of four fingers; assists in wrist flexion

sion occurs when the elbow is extended past this angle (Figure 14.14). It is created in large part by ligament laxity, and it is unlikely to change.

Another positional fault that can occur at the elbow joint is caused by the relationship of the ulna and the humerus and is called the carrying angle (Figure 14.15). The carrying angle has to do with the way the ulna is carried, or attached, to the humerus. It is more common in women.

The carrying angle can be observed when you flex your shoulders to 90 degrees, supinate your forearms, and place your fifth fingers together. There should be a straight line from the inner shoulder joint running distally to the medial wrist. If the elbows are inside this line or even touch during full extension of the elbow joint, then a carrying angle is present. An increased carrying angle can contribute to the instability of the elbow joint and is frequently found in conjunction with hyperextension.

Another structural aspect of the elbow joint is important to understand in order to prevent injury. In flexion of the elbow joint, the head of the radius is kept down in the radio-humeral joint by the healthy restriction of the annular ligament. During flexion and pronation at the radio-humeral

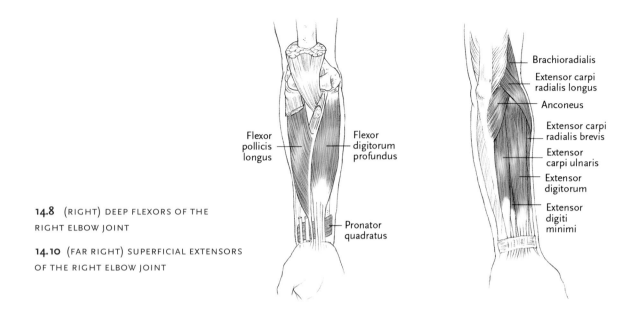

Flexor
pollicis
longus

Flexor
digitorum
profundus

Pronator
quadratus

Brachioradialis

Extensor carpi
radialis longus

Anconeus

Extensor carpi
radialis brevis

Extensor
carpi ulnaris

Extensor
digitorum

Extensor
digiti
minimi

14.8 (RIGHT) DEEP FLEXORS OF THE
RIGHT ELBOW JOINT

14.10 (FAR RIGHT) SUPERFICIAL EXTENSORS
OF THE RIGHT ELBOW JOINT

14.9 DEEP FLEXORS OF THE ELBOW JOINT

MUSCLE	ORIGIN	INSERTION	ACTION
Flexor digitorum profundus	Medial anterior ulna, interosseus membrane	Bases of distal phalanges of four fingers	Flexes distal phalanges of fingers; assists in wrist flexion
Flexor pollicis longus	Middle anterior radius, interosseus membrane	Distal phalanax of thumb	Flexes distal phalanx of thumb
Pronator quadratus	Distal ¼ of anterior ulna	Distal ¼ of anterior radius	Pronates arm

joint, the radius is being pulled upward by the biceps brachii. If you add to this strain by simultaneously lifting something heavy, it is possible to overstretch the annular ligament as the head of the radius moves up against it. Make sure that, when you make adjustments with students and when you carry props, you are careful not to strain this ligament in positions of pronation and flexion.

MUSCLE	ORIGIN	INSERTION	ACTION
Brachioradialis	Supracondylar ridge of humerus	Lateral styloid of radius	Flexes elbow with arm in neutral position
Extensor carpi radialis longus	Lateral supracondylar ridge of humerus, intermuscular septum	Radial side of second metacarpal bone	Extends and abducts wrist
Extensor carpi radialis brevis	Lateral epicondyle of humerus; common extensor tendon	Radial side of third metacarpal bone	Extends wrist
Extensor digitorum	Lateral epicondyle; common extensor tendon	Extensor expansions of medial four digits	Extends phalanges and wrist
Extensor digiti minimi	Lateral epicondyle; common extensor tendon	Extensor expansion of fifth finger	Extends fifth finger and wrist
Extensor carpi ulnaris	Lateral epicondyle; common extensor tendon	Base of the fifth metacarpal bone	Extends and abducts wrist
Anconeus	Lateral epicondyle of humerus; posterior ligament of elbow joint	Side of olecranon and posterior body of ulna	Assists triceps and extends elbow

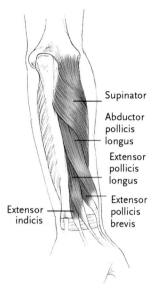

Supinator

Abductor
pollicis
longus

Extensor
pollicis
longus

Extensor
pollicis
brevis

Extensor
indicis

14.12 DEEP EXTENSORS OF THE RIGHT ELBOW JOINT

14.13 DEEP EXTENSORS OF THE ELBOW JOINT

MUSCLE	ORIGIN	INSERTION	ACTION
Supinator	Lateral epicondyle of humerus; proximal ulnar crest	Lateral proximal ⅓ of radius	Supinates hand
Abductor pollicis longus	Posterior radius; interosseus membrane	Base of first metacarpal	Abducts thumb; assists wrist abduction
Extensor pollicis longus	Posterior ulna; interosseus membrane	Base of distal phalanx of thumb	Extends distal phalanx of thumb; assists in wrist abduction
Extensor pollicis brevis	Flexor retinaculum; trapezium	First phalanx of thumb	Extends first metacarpal of thumb
Extensor indicis	Posterior ulna; interosseus membrane	Extensor digitorum of index finger	Extends proximal phalanx of index finger; assists in wrist extension

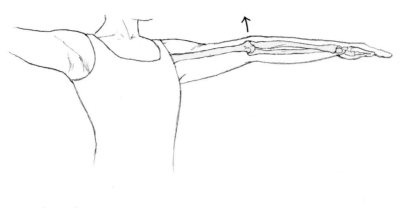

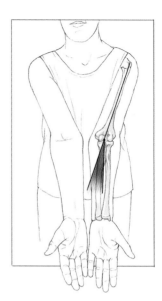

14.14 (ABOVE) HYPEREXTENDED ELBOW

14.15 (RIGHT) CARRYING ANGLE OF THE ELBOW

ESSENTIAL EXPERIENTIAL ANATOMY

For Practicing

14.16
ADHO MUKHA
SVANASANA

Applied Practice 1: Observing the Relationship of Hand and Elbow Position in Adho Mukha Svanasana

Prop: 1 nonskid mat

Take Care: Do not proceed if this pose causes discomfort in the elbow joints.

KNEEL ON your nonskid mat and, with an exhalation, lift up into Adho Mukha Svanasana (Figure 14.16). Place your hands so that your middle fingers point forward in the pose—in other words, your middle fingers are parallel to the edge of your mat. Now turn your fingers inward, and note the effect on the shoulder joints. Finally, try the pose with your fingers turning out.

Pay attention to the parallel relationship between the hands and shoulder joints. As your hands turn inward, so do the shoulder joints; as your hands turn outward, the shoulder joints rotate externally. This connection can be used to improve your shoulder function as well as to ameliorate pain in the elbows in the pose. By turning your hands outward in the pose, you can help to reduce the possibility of increasing hyperextension in the elbow joint.

Applied Practice 2: Observing the Position of the Elbow in Urdhva Dhanurasana

Prop: 1 nonskid mat

Take Care: Do not practice this pose during menstruation, after the first trimester of pregnancy, or if it causes lower back pain.

14.17
URDHVA
DHANURASANA

Lɪᴇ ᴏɴ your back on your nonskid mat. Bend your elbows, and place your hands on the mat so they are slightly wider than your shoulder joints (Figure 14.17). Turn your fingers about one-third of the way out. Make sure your elbows are held in. Often students place their hands close to the body, and then their elbows drop out. This decreases the power at the elbow joint as the elbow joints extend, because the triceps are no longer able to contract in the plane in which they lie when the elbows are not over the hands. Better to practice with the hands wider and the elbows narrower, rather than the opposite.

Now bend your knees, placing your feet next to your hips, with your feet turned inward. As you exhale, bring your lower back toward the floor and hold it there. With the next exhalation, push with your hands to move your pelvis in a diagonal direction up and out over your feet, and come up into the pose. Keep your breath even. Press your hands into the floor and, while not moving them, imagine that you are turning them out more, as if you were screwing them into the floor. This action of externally rotating the upper extremities with the hands fixed will help the scapula become fixed to the rib cage in such a way as to create more stability in the shoulder joint. Hold for up to 7 breaths and then come down. Repeat and experiment with the degree to which you turn your hands out.

14.18
SALAMBA
SIRSASANA,
LATERAL VIEW

Applied Practice 3: Elbow Position in Salamba Sirsasana
Prop: 1 nonskid mat
Take Care: Do not practice this preparatory pose during menstruation
or after the first trimester of pregnancy.
Fᴏʟᴅ ʏᴏᴜʀ ɴᴏɴꜱᴋɪᴅ ᴍᴀᴛ into fourths, and place it on a level surface. Get down on your hands and knees and prepare to place your arms down for Salamba Sirsasana (Figure 14.18), but do it in this very particular way. First place your right elbow on the mat, with your forearm perpendicular to the edge of the mat and your palm pointing toward the ceiling. Once you have placed you elbow on the mat, press down firmly and roll outward on this elbow. You will feel the skin and flesh around the elbow joint move. Do this same procedure with your left elbow.

Now keep your palms facing toward you (supination) and carefully lay your forearms down on the mat, so the tips of your fifth fingers touch and the forearms create a triangular shape. Again press firmly outward with your forearms, so you are resting fully along the shaft of the ulna. Now begin to pronate your forearms, so your thumbs point upward. Interlock your fingers, so your fifth fingers are not completely meshed at the base. This will help you keep your wrists perpendicular in the pose. Remember, the key bone is the distal radius; this is the focal point of awareness when you place your head into your hands for Salamba Sirsasana. This is the key bone to press against the head to keep the forearms active in the pose.

For Teaching

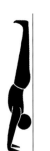

14.19

TADASANA,
ABDUCT THE UPPER
EXTREMITY AND
EXTEND THE ELBOW,
WITH THE PALMS
FACING UPWARD

Applied Teaching 1: Observing Hyperextension and the Carrying Angle of the Elbow Joint

Prop: 1 nonskid mat

Take Care: Do not force the elbow joint into hyperextension.

To OBSERVE the degree of hyperextension, if any, ask your student to perform the following. Have him abduct his upper extremity and extend the elbow fully with the palm facing upward (Figure 14.19). Now note the degree of extension. If past 180 degrees, hyperextension is present. This condition is more common in women.

What hyperextension means to asana practice is that, because of the relationship of the bones in hyperextension, the joint is a little more unstable. With hyperextension, the soft tissue and joint structure is allowing the bones to move past the point of maximum congruence on extension. When the joint surfaces are in maximum congruence, stability at the joint is also maximized. To create more elbow stability in Adho Mukha Vrksasana (Figure 14.20), ask your student to bend his elbows slightly to recreate a position of greater congruence.

14.20

ADHO MUKHA
VRKSASANA

Applied Teaching 2: Observing and Improving Hyperextension in Adho Mukha Vrksasana

Props: 1 nonskid mat • a wall

Take Care: Avoid this pose during menstruation, pregnancy, and up to three months postpartum.

As A TEACHER, you may know that students with hyperextended elbows have more difficulty with poses in which the elbow is bearing weight, such as Adho Mukha Vrksasana (Figure 14.20). When teaching this pose, attempt to create an alignment of 180 degrees at the elbow joint, even if the elbow feels a little bent to the practitioner. If the student is hyperextended in full extension, then flexing her elbows actually increases congruence at the joint surfaces.

Ask the student to practice the pose with the short side of a nonskid mat placed against a sturdy, smooth wall. When she is standing on her hands (and supported by the wall), make sure that her wrists, elbows, and shoulders are in one line. To do this, it may be necessary to have her slightly bend her elbows, or it may help to have her experiment with rotating her arms externally. Remember that hyperextension cannot be fixed but, through careful practice, students can avoid making it worse.

An injury to the elbow that is usually only seen in children is called a pulled elbow. This occurs when the head of the radius is pulled out of its annular ring, such as when the forearm is pulled or jerked suddenly. Symptoms include pain and difficulty in pronation and supination; flexion and extension are usually possible. For a full discussion of this injury, see *Caring for Your Baby and Young Child: Birth to Age Five* by Steven P. Shelov, M.D., and Robert E. Hannemann, M.D. (New York: Bantam, 2004). If you suspect this injury, consult a health care professional at once. To prevent it, remember to swing or playfully pull a child by both of his arms evenly, instead of by just one arm at a time.

The Wrist and Hand 15

LISTEN TO WHAT YOU KNOW THROUGH YOUR BODY.

—FRANCES PAYNE ADLER

ONE OF THE most important skills we can have as teachers is the ability to use our hands well. The awareness and intelligence we manifest as we gently touch and guide our students during class is at the heart of teaching compassionately. Likewise, learning how to guide our students as they strengthen their wrists and hands is a valuable gift to impart. It can improve their practice and protect them from possible injury.

BONES

The eight wrist bones are called in the aggregate the carpals or carpal bones. Viewing the two rows of carpals in the anatomical position (palmar view), the proximal row, from lateral (thumb side) to medial, consists of the scaphoid, the lunate, the triquetral, and the pisiform bones. The scaphoid and lunate bones articulate with the distal end of the radius. The distal row of carpals, from lateral to medial, are the trapezium, the trapezoid, the capitate, and the hamate bones. The distal row of carpal bones articulates with the metacarpal bones of the hand.

One way to remember the order and names of the carpals is to memorize this phrase: "Some lovers try positions that they can't handle." The first letters of the eight carpal bones (Figure 15.1), from lateral to medial, are the same as the first letters of the words of this sentence. Figure 15.2 describes the carpals individually.

Practice palpating the proximal row of carpals. Have a student present the posterior surface of her left hand. After asking permission to touch her, find the proximal end of the first metacarpal bone at the radial styloid side of the hand. Now move just proximally to palpate the trapezium bone. Then move your fingers laterally to find the trapezoid bone. Next over you will feel a depression under your fingers; this is the capitate bone. Passively flex and extend the student's wrist. One

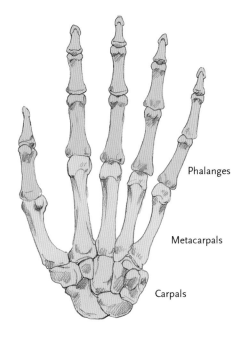

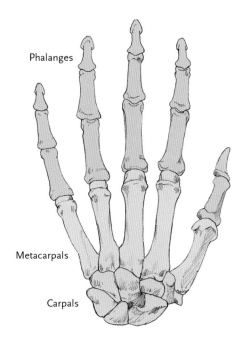

Phalanges

Metacarpals

Carpals

15.1 (ABOVE LEFT) CARPALS, METACARPALS, AND PHA-
LANGES OF THE LEFT HAND, ANTERIOR (PALMAR) VIEW

15.3 (ABOVE RIGHT) CARPALS, METACARPALS, AND
PHALANGES OF THE LEFT HAND, POSTERIOR VIEW

more bone over is the hamate. Try palpating the
palmar surface of this bone at the same time; see
if you can feel the hook of the hamate on the palmar side. Do this by putting your right thumb on
the posterior surface of the hamate and your right
index finger on the palmar hook of the bone. The
next bone is the triquetral bone. The pisiform sits
on the palmar side of the triquetral, distal to the
hamate (Figure 15.3).

The bones of the hand proper are the metacarpals. The metacarpals are the long slender bones
of the body of the hand and are numbered from
the thumb to the fifth finger. The metacarpals consist of a body, a base at the proximal side for articulation with the carpals, and a rounded head that
articulates with the proximal phalanx.

The phalanges consist of three segments: a proximal, a medial, and a distal, except the thumb, which
has only two segments, a proximal and a distal.

Joints

Few joint bones have as complex a relationship
with each other as the carpals. They articulate with
the radius and with each other at myriad joints. It
is usual to omit the ulna as articulating with the
carpals, as it technically articulates with an articular disc.

Note that, while the metacarpals are in full flexion, the interossei muscles cannot perform adduction or abduction. Try this for yourself. Extend
your fingers fully, and try abducting and adduct-
ing them. It is easy. Now fully flex your fingers; you
will be unable to either adduct or abduct them. (See
Figure 15.9 for more information on the interossei muscles.) The interrosei are at a biomechanical
disadvantage to adduct or abduct the joints in full
flexion because the muscles are stretched and thus
weakened in this position.

The interphalangeal (IP) joints are much more
limited than the metacarpal joints. The IP joints are
only able to flex and extend. The former movement
is much greater in range; the latter movement is
limited by ligaments.

BONE	LOCATION/DESCRIPTION	ARTICULATIONS
Scaphoid	Boat-shaped; largest and most lateral of proximal row; frequently fractured by hyperextension and abduction of wrist	Radius distally, trapezium, trapezoid medially, capitate, and lunate
Lunate	Crescent-shaped; head of capitate articulates with hollow of crescent	Radius proximally and articular disk, scaphoid laterally, capitate, hamate, medially triquetral
Triquetral	Pyramidal shape; most medial bone in proximal row; distal to pisiform	Lunate proximally, pisiform and hamate; articular disk
Pisiform	Small size and easily palpable; protects tendon of flexor carpi ulnaris muscle by bearing force generated by tendon riding across triquetral bone, especially during wrist extension	Triquetral
Trapezium	Most lateral carpal bone in distal row; forms saddle joint with first metacarpal (thumb)	Scaphoid, first and second metacarpals, and trapezoid
Trapezoid	Smallest bone in distal row; trapezoid shape	Scaphoid, second metacarpal laterally, trapezium, capitate medially
Capitate	Largest carpal; located in center of wrist	Scaphoid proximally, lunate, trapezoid, hamate medially; second, third, and fourth metacarpals
Hamate	Most medial carpal bone in distal row; hook-shaped process on palmar surface	Lunate laterally, medially and proximally to the triquetral; capitate laterally; fourth and fifth metacarpals

CONNECTIVE TISSUE

The ligamentous structure of the wrist, carpals, and metacarpals is complex and outside the scope of this book. To learn more, please consult *Gray's Anatomy*. But some information about the connective tissue of the wrist can be interesting to yoga teachers. One structure that is important to understand is the retinaculum, a thickened band of connective tissue, which is shaped like a cuff that surrounds the wrist joint (Figure 15.4). It holds the long tendons around the wrist close to the bone and has two parts. The anterior part is called the flexor retinaculum and is made up of two bands, the palmar carpal ligament and the transverse carpal ligament, which is deeper and more distal. The second part is the extensor retinaculum on the posterior side. It runs from the styloid process to the lateral margin of the radius.

NERVES

The nerves to the wrist joint arise from the ulnar nerve and from the dorsal interosseous nerve (Figure 15.4). One of the common problems with nerves at the wrist is carpal tunnel syndrome (CTS), or repetitive stress injury (RSI). This is irritation of the median nerve as it passes the wrist. Here's how it happens.

An arch is formed by the carpal bones and the transverse carpal ligament that is part of the flexor retinaculum. This arch is called the carpal tunnel. The tendons of the flexor digitorum profundus and superficialis, the flexor carpi radialis, and the flexor pollicis longus pass under the retinaculum here. Additionally the median nerve passes through this arched tunnel. Remember that that the flexor retinaculum restricts the bowing of the long flexor tendons and protects the median nerve here.

RSI is created by repeated ischemic insults to the median nerve from repeated extension of the wrist while the fingers are in flexion. This is exactly the position of the wrist and hand during computer work, when one is typing and using the mouse. Some cases of RSI can be helped by stretching gently in the other direction, that is, flexion of the wrist and simultaneous extension of the fingers. If you guess that your student suffers from RSI, send him to a health care professional for diagnosis and deep tissue work to relieve the compression.

MUSCLES

The wrist proper has no intrinsic muscles. Rather, the wrist is controlled by the muscles originating on the forearm. These muscles are presented in chapter 14.

15.4 (BELOW LEFT) FLEXOR RETINACULUM AND NERVES TO THE WRIST

15.5 (BELOW RIGHT) MUSCLES OF THE THENAR EMINENCE

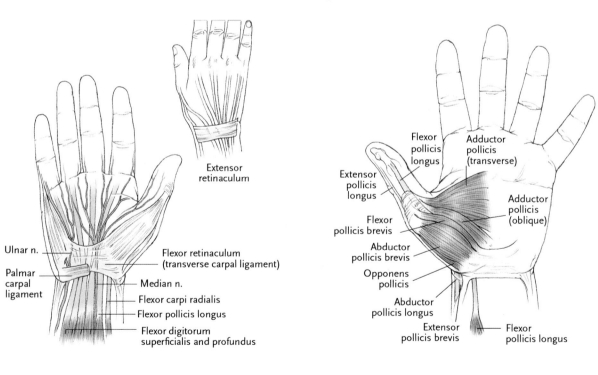

Extensor retinaculum

Ulnar n.

Palmar carpal ligament

Flexor retinaculum (transverse carpal ligament)

Median n.

Flexor carpi radialis

Flexor pollicis longus

Flexor digitorum superficialis and profundus

Flexor pollicis longus

Adductor pollicis (transverse)

Extensor pollicis longus

Adductor pollicis (oblique)

Flexor pollicis brevis

Abductor pollicis brevis

Opponens pollicis

Abductor pollicis longus

Extensor pollicis brevis

Flexor pollicis longus

MUSCLE	ORIGIN	INSERTION	ACTION
Abductor pollicis longus	Anterior radius, ulna, interosseous membranes	Distal phalanx of first metacarpal	Flexes distal phalanx
Abductor pollicis brevis	Flexor retinaculum	Proximal phalanx of thumb, near flexor pollicis brevis	Abducts and medially rotates thumb
Opponens pollicis	Trapezium and flexor retinaculum	Metacarpal of thumb	Abducts, flexes, and rotates metacarpal of thumb
Flexor pollicis longus	Anterior radius and interosseus membrane	Distal phalanx of thumb	Flexes distal phalanx
Flexor pollicis brevis	Radius and interosseous membrane	Base of the proximal phalanx of thumb	Extends proximal phalanx of thumb; assists wrist abduction
Extensor pollicis longus	Posterior ulna and interosseous membrane	Base of distal phalanx of thumb	Extends interphalangeal joint
Extensor pollicis brevis	Posterior radius and interosseous membrane	Base of proximal phalanx of thumb; tendon under extensor retinaculum	Extends metacarpal and carpo-metacarpal joints of thumb
Adductor pollicis	Capitate trapezoid, trapezium, second and third metacarpals	Medial base of proximal phalanx of thumb; metacarpal phalangeal joint	Adducts thumb

The muscles of the hand are divided into three groups. The first group is the muscles of the thumb (pollex), which collectively form the thenar eminence (Figures 15.5 and 15.6). At the opposite side of the hand are the hypothenar muscles (Figures 15.7 and 15.8). The term *digiti minimi* refers to the "small digit," or fifth finger. The final set of hand muscles is called the intermediate muscles (Figure 15.9).

KINESIOLOGY

Under normal circumstances, the wrist and hand are not weight-bearing structures. But in asana class, they sometimes bear weight in poses like Chaturanga Dandasana and Adho Mukha Vrksasana. There are two ways of keeping the wrists and hands healthy; one is by strengthening the forearm muscles, and the other is by paying atten-

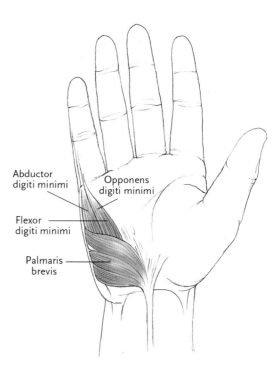

15.7 MUSCLES OF THE HYPOTHENAR EMINENCE

Abductor digiti minimi

Opponens digiti minimi

Flexor digiti minimi

Palmaris brevis

tion to the alignment of the hands, especially, during weight bearing.

To keep the wrists strong, you must keep the forearm muscles, both extensors and flexors, strong. This can be done by simple resistive exercises using hand weights under the guidance of a qualified trainer.

To prevent wrist injury, pay attention to the placement of the hands on the floor in weight bearing. This is especially true for poses like Adho Mukha Vrksasana and Bakasana, when all the weight of the body is borne directly down onto the wrists. For more details on proper technique, see the Applied Teaching section in this chapter.

It is a well-known kinesiological principle that, in order to stretch the flexors of a joint, the extensors must contract, and vice versa. This is true of the wrist and hand, of course, but it is also illustrated by a special effect on the extensor tendons of the hand and wrist in flexion, called tendon fixation or binding effect. This is how it works.

Make a fist with one hand, and then fully flex that same wrist. Now, keeping the hand well flexed, use your other hand to attempt to push your fist into deeper flexion. Take care to do this slowly to avoid injury. You will find that your fingers will uncurl and extend, even while your wrist remains flexed. This is because the long extensor muscles of the wrist and fingers are overstretched by the extreme flexion you are creating. Therefore these tendons attempt to protect themselves by overriding the flexors and producing extension.

The same effect can be seen in extension of the wrist. Once again, make a strong closed fist with one hand, and then extend that wrist. Now use your other hand to attempt to pry open the fingers of the closely held flexed fist, while you keep your wrist in extension. Once again, proceed with care. With the help of your other hand, you will find that it becomes easy to open the fingers of the fist. The fingers open more easily than when the wrist is in flexion; this occurs to protect the long flexors of the wrist from being overstretched during forced wrist extension.

15.8 Muscles of the Hypothenar Eminence

Muscle	Origin	Insertion	Action
Palmaris brevis	Transverse carpal ligament	Skin on ulnar border of palm	Draws skin at ulnar side of palm toward middle of palm
Abductor digiti minimi	Pisiform bone	Ulnar side of proximal phalanx of fifth finger	Abducts fifth finger and flexes proximal phalanx
Flexor digiti minimi brevis	Hook of hamate bone and flexor retinaculum	Proximal phalanx of fifth finger	Flexes proximal phalanx of metacarpal-phalangeal joint of fifth finger
Opponens digiti minimi	Hook of hamate bone and flexor retinaculum	Ulnar side of fifth metacarpal bone of fifth finger	Abducts, flexes, and rotates fifth metacarpal

15.9 Intermediate Muscles of the Hand

Muscle	Origin	Insertion	Action
Lumbricales	Flexor digitorum profundus tendons	Extensor expansion of extensor digitorum; second, third, fourth, and fifth proximal phalanges	Flex metacarpal-phalangeal joints (MP) and extend two distal phalanges (PIP and DIP)
Interossei	Two heads, adjacent to dorsal and palmar metacarpals	Sides of the proximal phalanges to extensor expansion of the dorsal second, third, and fourth fingers, and palmar surface of second, fourth, and fifth fingers	Posterior (dorsal) portions abduct fingers; anterior (palmar) adducts phalanges

Experiential Anatomy

For Practicing

15.10
VIRASANA,
WITH HANDS
IN FRONT OF
THE FACE

Applied Practice 1: Stretching the Flexors of the Wrist

Prop: 1 nonskid mat or a chair

Take Care: Avoid sitting in Virasana if it is uncomfortable for your knees;
practice sitting in a chair instead.

Sɪᴛ ɪɴ Vɪʀᴀsᴀɴᴀ on your nonskid mat or a chair (Figure 15.10). Place your hands in front of your face with your palms facing you. Bring the outer edges of the hands together, so the fifth fingers are touching. Now lean forward and put your hands on the floor, with the fingers facing toward you, the insides of the wrists pointing away, and the palms flat on the floor. The cubital fossa of the elbow is facing outward, and the olecranon is facing toward you; the thumbs are on the outside, fifth fingers on the inside.

Now lean back, as if to sit in Virasana, while keeping your hands on the floor. This will cause a strong stretch of your flexors. Hold the stretch for 3 to 5 breaths, rest, and then repeat.

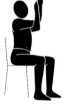

15.11
SEATED WRIST
EXTENSOR
STRETCH

Applied Practice 2: Stretching the Extensors of the Wrist

Prop: 1 nonskid mat or a chair

Take Care: Avoid this pose if it causes pain in the wrist.

Tʜɪs ᴍᴀʏ seem a little complicated but it is worth the trouble. Begin by sitting in a comfortable position with your arms straight in front of you (shoulder flexion). Cross your left wrist over your right. Now turn your palms so they are facing each other and pressed together, and interlock your fingers (Figure 15.11). Be sure to keep your palms firmly together.

Inhale, and as you exhale, pull up and backwards on your left hand, so you can see the back of that hand completely and it moves closer to your face. You will likely feel a strong but pleasant stretch in the extensors of your right forearm. To increase that stretch, keep the traction of the stretch and internally rotate your right arm, so the back of your right hand faces the floor. Remember to breathe while you practice. Repeat twice on each side.

For Teaching

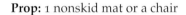

Applied Teaching 1: Hand Position in Adho Mukha Vrksasana

Prop: 1 nonskid mat

Take Care: Avoid this pose during pregnancy or menstruation;
if you have glaucoma, retinal problems, hiatal hernia, or a wrist injury;
or if you are more than thirty pounds overweight.

Mᴀɴʏ sᴛᴜᴅᴇɴᴛs are taught to flatten the palm against the floor when they practice Adho Mukha Vrksasana (Figure 15.12). But that may not be the healthiest position. To under-

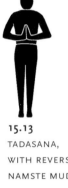

15.12
ADHO MUKHA
VRKSASANA

stand why, first note that the foot has three main arches to facilitate weight bearing. It makes sense then that, especially for a structure that is not normally weight bearing, like the wrist, it would be beneficial to create an arch there as well.

Have your student try this experiment. Ask her to get down onto her hands and knees on the mat and place her palms flat on the floor, directly under her shoulders, and then lean forward. She will very likely feel some compression in the extensor side of her wrists. After releasing this attempt, ask her to place her hands on the mat once again and then slide back the tips of her fingers slightly, to create an arch in the palm. Have her lean forward. The weight will now be disbursed throughout her hand, and her wrist will feel much better.

In this position, the edges of the hand are touching the floor, but the middle of the palm is not. This position will protect the wrist as well as engage the intrinsic muscles of the fingers and hand in a way that adds support to the area. Now have her move her mat to the wall and try Adho Mukha Vrksasana to experience the pose with weight bearing on the edges of the hand and an inner arch.

15.13
TADASANA,
WITH REVERSE
NAMSTE MUDRA

Applied Teaching 2: Reverse Namaste Mudra
Prop: 1 nonskid mat
Take Care: Avoid this pose if you have a wrist injury.

HAVE YOUR STUDENT practice Tadasana on a nonskid mat. Instruct him to abduct his right arm and bring it behind his back. Suggest that he reach across with his left hand to help move the right hand and arm up the back. Now bring the left hand onto the back. With an exhalation, have him slide both hands up his back near the spinal column, with the palms facing outward. With an exhalation, have him externally rotate his upper arms, drop the elbows and shoulder blades, and then slowly turn his hands and press them, palm to palm, in the Namaste mudra. Hold for several breaths, release, and repeat.

LINK

A mudra is a seal that is intended to hold or direct energy in the body. The next time you teach Savasana, have your students take Gyan mudra. First suggest that your students have their arms out to the side in a comfortable position, with the palms turned upward. Now practice the mudra by placing the tip of the index finger just at the base of the distal phalangeal joint of the thumb, so the index finger is caught by the natural curve of the thumb as the hand relaxes in the pose. There should be no effort expended in keeping the mudra. The hand continues to be at ease, with the other fingers gently curled. In this mudra, the index finger represents the individual, and the thumb represents the universal. This mudra expresses their union and serves to bring attention inward in the pose.

About the Author

A YOGA TEACHER since 1971, Judith Hanson Lasater holds a bachelor of science degree in physical therapy from the University of California, San Francisco, as well as a doctorate in East-West psychology from the California Institute of Integral Studies. In 1974 she helped found the Institute for Yoga Teacher Education (now the Iyengar Institute of San Francisco), a nationally known yoga teacher training program that has since trained thousands of teachers.

In 1975 she cofounded *Yoga Journal* magazine. Judith modeled yoga poses for *Yoga Journal* and started and served on its editorial advisory board. She created and wrote the asana column in the magazine for thirteen years, as well as dozens of other articles relating to postures, anatomy, kinesiology, yoga therapeutics, breathing exercises, and the psychology and philosophy of yoga. She continues to write regularly for *Yoga Journal* as a nationally recognized authority on yoga and serves on the magazine's advisory board.

She is president of the California Yoga Teachers Association, the oldest independent professional yoga teachers association in the United States, with over 6,000 members. She has served on the advisory boards of the International Yoga Studies Association, the medical journal *Alternative Thera-pies*, and the national registry association for yoga teachers, Yoga Alliance.

Judith has taught yoga as an invited teacher at national and international conventions of yoga teachers for decades. For three years she was a featured speaker at the Governor's Women's Conference in Long Beach, CA, and was the opening keynote speaker at *Yoga Journal*'s annual yoga conference. She has also been a speaker at the IDEA-*Yoga Journal* Conference in Anaheim, CA, the Yoga Northwest Conference, the Kripalu Conscious Parenting Conference, and the Yoga in Toronto Conference.

She has trained beginning students and teachers alike in asana, pranayama (breathing), meditation, anatomy, kinesiology, yoga therapeutics, yoga philosophy, and restorative yoga, one of her specialties. She teaches in San Francisco as well as across the United States and throughout the world. During her second visit to Russia, she directed the production of a video on therapeutic yoga to be used in Russian military hospitals. She has also been an invited guest teacher for the heart patients in Dr. Dean Ornish's Preventative Health program for heart disease as well as in his prostate study using yoga. In 2007 she was an invited speaker at UC Davis School of Medicine, under the auspices of the Complimentary and Alternative Medicine Program.

Judith is the author of:

Relax and Renew (1995)
Living Your Yoga (2000)
30 Essential Yoga Poses (2003)
Yoga for Pregnancy (2004)
Yoga Abs (2005)
A Year of Living Your Yoga (2006)
Yogabody (2009)
What We Say Matters (2009)

Judith is currently writing a regular feature called "Real Yoga" for *Yoga Journal* magazine. She also acts as a health and movement consultant for several other national magazines, including *Shape*, *Men's Health*, and *Body + Soul*. She has served as an advisor for a National Institutes of Health (NIH) project studying the effects of yoga on lower back pain for the Osher Center for Integrative Medicine, as well as a consultant on another NIH project on chronic obstructive pulmonary disease (COPD) with the University of San Francisco. She recently completed advising an NIH study using restorative yoga to reduce hot flashes and is consulting on two other NIH studies, one on pregnancy and restorative yoga and another on restorative yoga for reducing anxiety for participants in drug rehabilitation.

She lives in the San Francisco Bay Area. For more information about her yoga classes and teleclasses, workshops, retreats, and teacher trainings, visit www.judithlasater.com and www.restorativeyogateachers.com.

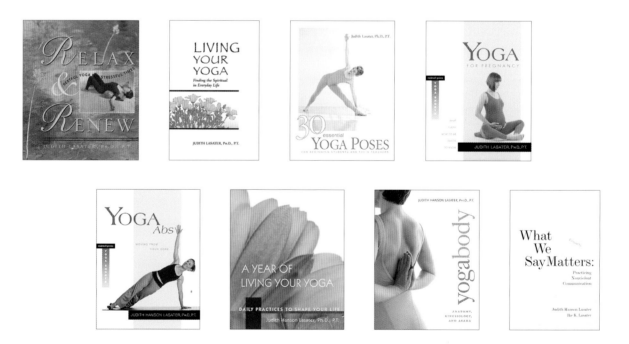

From the Publisher

RODMELL PRESS publishes books on yoga, Buddhism, aikido, and Taoism. In the Bhagavadgita it is written, "Yoga is skill in action." It is our hope that our books will help individuals develop a more skillful practice—one that brings peace to their daily lives and to the earth.

We thank those whose support, encouragement, and practical advice sustain us in our efforts. In particular, we are grateful to Reb Anderson, B. K. S. Iyengar, Wendy Palmer, and Yvonne Rand for their inspiration.

CATALOG REQUEST

(510) 841-3123 or (800) 841-3123
(510) 841-3123 (fax)
info@rodmellpress.com
www.rodmellpress.com

TRADE SALES/UNITED STATES, INTERNATIONAL

Publishers Group West
(800) 788-3123
(510) 528-5511 (sales fax)
info@pgw.com
www.pgw.com

FOREIGN LANGUAGE AND BOOK CLUB RIGHTS

Linda Cogozzo, Publisher
(510) 841-3123
linda@rodmellpress.com
www.rodmellpress.com

Index